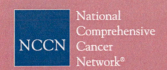

NCCN Guidelines for Patients®
Version 1.2016

Breast Cancer
Early-Stage
STAGES I AND II

NCCN Foundation® gratefully acknowledges:

Support from

NCCN AND NCCN FOUNDATION – BOARDS OF DIRECTORS
Drs. Al B. Benson III and Alanah Fitch
Joshua and Stephanie Bilenker
Dr. and Mrs. Douglas W. Blayney
Mara Bloom
Rebecca Caires, MBA
Peter F. Coccia, MD and Phyllis I. Warkentin, MD
Gena Cook
Dr. and Mrs. Thomas A. D'Amico
Dr. and Mrs. Timothy J. Eberlein
Paul F. Engstrom
David S. Ettinger, MD, FACP, FCCP
Theresa J. Franco, RN, MSN
Brian Garofalo
Jack A. Gentile, Jr.
Matt Kalaycio, MD
Mark F. Kochevar and Barbara Redmond
Heather Kopecky
Trisha Lollo
Ray Lynch, CPA, MBA
James and Marilyn Mohler
Lisle M. Nabell, MD
Michael and Gwyneth Neuss
Michael Parisi, MBA, MA
Barbara Parker, MD
Lori C Pickens, MHA
Dorothy Puhy
Denise K. Reinke, MS, NP
Marc Samuels
Gerrie Shields
Dr. and Mrs. Samuel Silver
Susan C. & Robert P. Stein
The Honorable Ellen O. Tauscher
Jeff and Colleen Walker
Robert C. Young, MD

NCCN AND NCCN FOUNDATION – STAFF CONTRIBUTING $100 OR MORE
Anonymous
Robert W. Carlson, MD and Stacey Starcher
C. Lyn Fitzgerald, MJ
Kristina Gregory
Joseph Junod

Lisa G. Kimbro, MBA, CPA
Joan S. McClure
Elizabeth Nardi
Marcie Reeder, MPH
Gary J. and Marianne Weyhmuller

An additional fifty-five (55) donations were received from other NCCN staff members.

Endorsed by

BREAST CANCER ALLIANCE
Receiving a cancer diagnosis can be overwhelming, both for the patient and their family. We support the NCCN guidelines for breast cancer with the knowledge that these tools will help to equip patients with many of the educational resources, and answers to questions, they may seek. www.breastcanceralliance.org

FORCE: FACING OUR RISK OF CANCER EMPOWERED
As the nation's leading organization serving the hereditary breast and ovarian cancer community, FORCE is pleased to endorse the NCCN Guidelines for Patients with breast cancer. This guide provides valuable, evidence-based, expert-reviewed information on the standard of care, empowering patients to make informed decisions about their treatment. www.facingourrisk.org

LIVING BEYOND BREAST CANCER
Receiving a diagnosis of breast cancer is overwhelming. Having trusted information is essential to help understand one's particular diagnosis and treatment options. The information found in the NCCN Guidelines for Patients: Breast Cancer is accessible, accurate, and will help every step of the way—from the moment of diagnosis through treatment. People can use the NCCN Guidelines for Patients: Breast Cancer to become an informed partner in their own care.
www.lbbc.org

SHARSHERET
Sharsheret is proud to endorse this important resource, the NCCN Guidelines for Patients: Breast Cancer. With this critical tool in hand, women nationwide have the knowledge they need to partner with their healthcare team to navigate the often complicated world of breast cancer care and make informed treatment decisions. www.sharsheret.org

YOUNG SURVIVAL COALITION (YSC)
Young Survival Coalition (YSC) is pleased to endorse the NCCN Guidelines for Patients: Breast Cancer as an invaluable resource for young women diagnosed with breast cancer and their co-survivors. This in-depth, illustrated series clearly explains what breast cancer is, how it is treated and what patients can expect on the journey ahead. www.youngsurvival.org

Special thank you to

ROCKIN' FOR THE CURE®
NCCN Foundation would like to thank Rockin' for the Cure for providing much needed support for the NCCN Guidelines for Patients! Rockin' For The Cure 2016 was a giant success and we are incredibly grateful to the Rockin' For The Cure team for their hard work and passion to promote cancer awareness. We look forward to 2017.
www.rockinforthecure.net

Credits

NCCN aims to improve the care given to patients with cancer. NCCN staff work with experts to create helpful programs and resources for many stakeholders. Stakeholders include health providers, patients, businesses, and others. One resource is the series of books for patients called the NCCN Guidelines for Patients®. Each book presents the best practice for a type of cancer. The patient books are based on clinical practice guidelines written for cancer doctors. These guidelines are called the NCCN Clinical Practice Guidelines in Oncology (NCCN Guidelines®). Clinical practice guidelines list the best health care options for groups of patients. Many doctors use them to help plan cancer treatment for their patients.

Panels of experts create the NCCN Guidelines®. Most of the experts are from NCCN Member Institutions. Panelists may include surgeons, radiation oncologists, medical oncologists, and patient advocates. Recommendations in the NCCN Guidelines are based on clinical trials and the experience of the panelists. The NCCN Guidelines are updated at least once a year. When funded, the patient books are updated to reflect the most recent version of the NCCN Guidelines for doctors. For more information about the NCCN Guidelines, visit NCCN.org/clinical.asp.

NCCN staff involved in developing the NCCN Guidelines for Patients include:

Dorothy A. Shead, MS
Director, Patient and Clinical Information Operations

Laura J. Hanisch, PsyD
Medical Writer/Patient Information Specialist

Lacey Marlow
Associate Medical Writer

Rachael Clarke
Guidelines Data and Layout Coordinator

Susan Kidney
Graphic Design Specialist

Supported by NCCN Foundation®

NCCN Foundation supports the mission of the National Comprehensive Cancer Network® (NCCN®) to improve the care of patients with cancer. One of its aims is to raise funds to create a library of books for patients. Learn more about the NCCN Foundation at NCCN.org/foundation.

National Comprehensive Cancer Network (NCCN)
275 Commerce Drive • Suite 300
Fort Washington, PA 19034
215.690.0300

© 2016 National Comprehensive Cancer Network, Inc. All rights reserved.
The NCCN Guidelines for Patients® and illustrations herein may not be reproduced in any form for any purpose without the express written permission of NCCN.

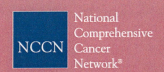

NCCN Guidelines for Patients® Version 1.2016

Breast Cancer
Early-Stage

STAGES I AND II

Breast cancer is the most common type of cancer in women. Learning that you have breast cancer can feel overwhelming. The goal of this book is to help you get the best care. It presents which cancer tests and treatments for stages I and II breast cancer are recommended by experts.

The National Comprehensive Cancer Network® (NCCN®) is a not-for-profit alliance of 27 of the world's leading cancer centers. Experts from NCCN have written treatment guidelines for doctors who treat breast cancer. These treatment guidelines suggest what the best practice is for cancer care. The information in this patient book is based on the guidelines written for doctors.

This book focuses on the treatment of stages I & II breast cancer. Key points of the book are summarized in the related **NCCN Quick Guide™**. NCCN also offers patient resources on stages 0, III, and IV breast cancer, ovarian cancer, sarcoma, lymphomas, and other cancer types. Visit **NCCN.org/patients** for the full library of patient books, summaries, and other patient and caregiver resources.

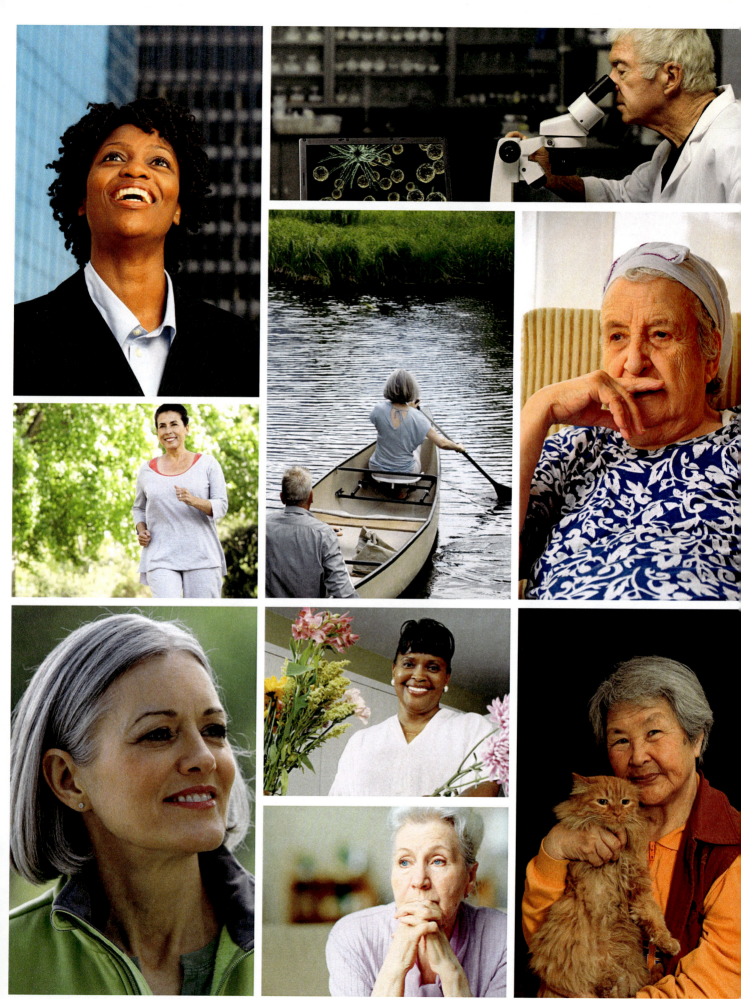

Contents

Breast Cancer
Early-Stage
STAGES I AND II

4 How to use this book

5 **Part 1**
Breast cancer basics
Explains breast cancer and its treatment.

15 **Part 2**
Treatment planning
Describes how doctors plan your treatment.

27 **Part 3**
Breast cancer surgery
Presents your options for removing the cancer and rebuilding breasts.

39 **Part 4**
Chemotherapy and HER2 inhibitors
Presents if these cancer drugs may be right for you.

55 **Part 5**
Radiation therapy
Presents if you may need this treatment and to which body sites.

65 **Part 6**
Endocrine therapy
Presents if you may need this treatment and which type.

75 **Part 7**
Follow-up care
Presents key parts of long-term health care.

81 **Part 8**
Breast cancer recurrence
Presents your treatment options if the cancer returns.

87 **Part 9**
Making treatment decisions
Offers tips for choosing the best treatment.

95 Glossary:
96 Dictionary
100 Acronyms

103 NCCN Panel Members

104 NCCN Member Institutions

106 Index

How to use this book

Who should read this book?

This book is about treatment for stages I and II breast cancer among women. Patients and those who support them—caregivers, family, and friends—may find this book helpful. It may help you discuss and decide with doctors what care is best.

Where should I start reading?

Starting with Part 1 may be helpful. It explains what stages I and II breast cancer is. Understanding the cancer will help you understand its treatment. An overview of treatment options is also given.

Part 2 lists what health care is needed before treatment. Some types of health care help your doctors plan treatment. Other health care can address health issues beyond cancer treatment.

Parts 3 through 7 are a step-by-step guide to your treatment options. Options are based on the best science that exists for stages I and II breast cancer. Part 8 lists key parts to your health care once you are cancer-free. Part 9 offers some helpful tips on getting the best care.

Does the whole book apply to me?

This book includes information for many situations. Your treatment team can help. They can point out what information applies to you. They can also give you more information. As you read through this book, you may find it helpful to make a list of questions to ask your doctors.

The recommendations in this book are based on science and the experience of NCCN experts. However, these recommendations may not be right for you. Your doctors may suggest other tests and treatments based on your health and other factors. If other recommendations are given, feel free to ask your treatment team questions.

Making sense of medical terms

In this book, many medical words are included. These are words that you will likely hear from your treatment team. Most of these words may be new to you, and it may be a lot to learn.

Don't be discouraged as you read. Keep reading and review the information. Don't be shy to ask your treatment team to explain a word or phrase that you do not understand.

Words that you may not know are defined in the text or in the *Dictionary*. Words in the *Dictionary* are underlined when first used on a page.

Acronyms are also defined when first used and in the *Glossary*. Acronyms are short words formed from the first letters of several words. One example is DNA for **d**eoxyribo**n**ucleic **a**cid.

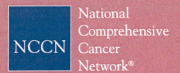

1
Breast cancer basics

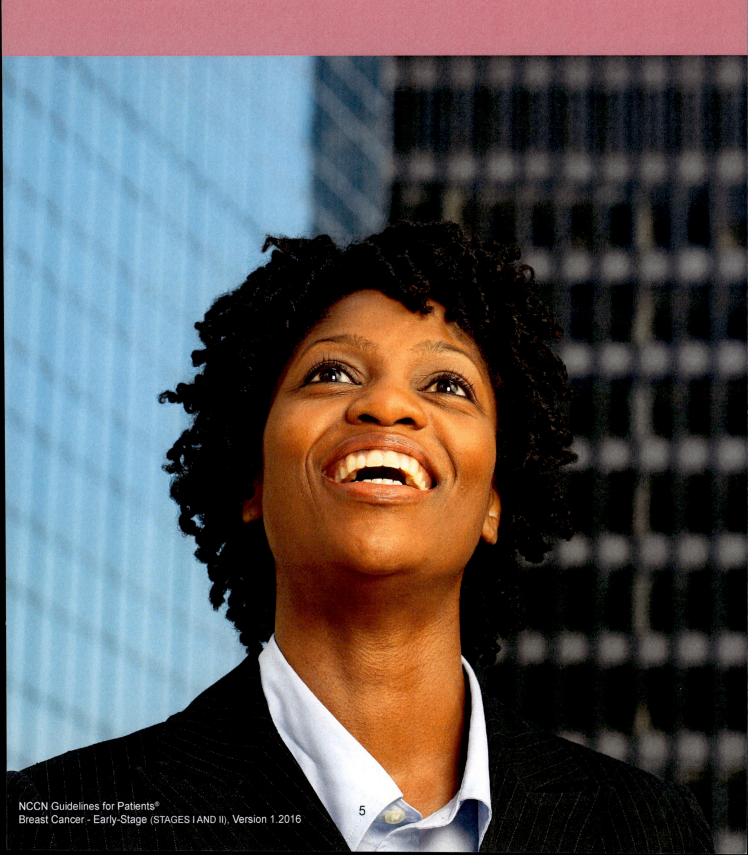

1 Breast cancer basics

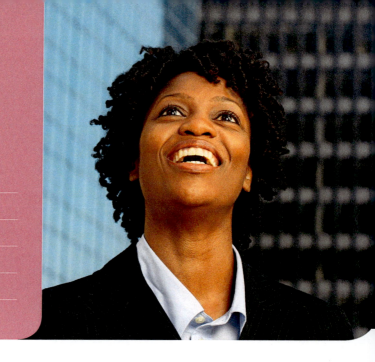

6   Women's breasts
8   Breast cancer
10 Cancer stage
10 Treatment options
14 Review

You've learned that you have breast cancer. It's common to feel shocked and confused. Part 1 reviews some basics that may help you learn about breast cancer and its treatment.

Women's breasts

Before learning about breast cancer, it is helpful to know about breasts. The ring of darker skin seen on the outside of the breast is called the areola. The raised tip in the middle of the areola is called the nipple. In young girls, there are small ducts under the nipple that branch into fatty tissue like early growth from a seedling. These immature ducts are supported by connective tissue called stroma.

Increases in female hormones among girls during puberty cause their breasts to change. The stroma increases, the ducts grow and branch out like tree limbs, and lobules form at the end of the ducts like leaves at the end of twigs. Lobules are small sacs that make breast milk after a baby is born. Breast milk drains from the millions of leaf-like lobules into the ducts that connect to the nipple. **See Figure 1.1** for a look inside women's breasts.

Lymph is a clear fluid that gives cells water and food and helps to fight germs. It drains from breast tissue into lymph vessels within the stroma. **See Figure 1.2**. Then, it travels to the breast's lymph nodes, most of which are in your armpit. Lymph nodes are small structures that filter and remove germs from lymph. Nodes near the armpit are called axillary lymph nodes.

1 Breast cancer basics | Women's breasts

Figure 1.1
Inside women's breasts

Inside of women's breasts are millions of lobules that form breast milk after a baby is born. Breast milk drains from the lobules into ducts that carry the milk to the nipple. Around the lobules and ducts is soft tissue called stroma.

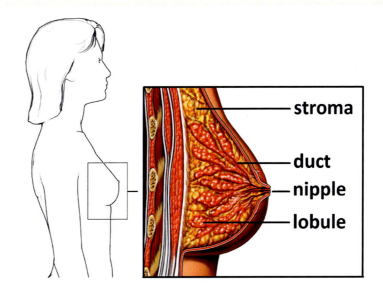

Illustration Copyright © 2016 Nucleus Medical Media, All rights reserved. www.nucleusinc.com

Figure 1.2
Breast lymph vessels and nodes

Lymph is a clear fluid that gives cells water and food and helps to fight germs. It drains from breast tissue into lymph vessels within the stroma. It then travels to the breast's lymph nodes, most of which are in the armpit ("axilla").

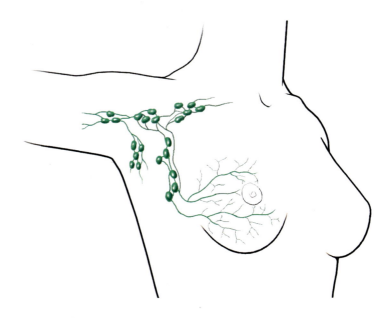

Illustration Copyright © 2016 Nucleus Medical Media, All rights reserved. www.nucleusinc.com

1 Breast cancer basics | Breast cancer

Breast cancer

Cancer is a disease of cells. Carcinomas are cancers of cells that make up the skin and the tissue that lines or covers organs. Almost all breast cancers are carcinomas. In the breast, carcinomas start in the cells lining either the ducts or lobules, but most breast cancers start in ductal cells.

Inside of cells are coded instructions for building new cells and controlling how cells behave. These instructions are called genes. Genes are a part of DNA (**d**eoxyribo**n**ucleic **a**cid), which is grouped together into bundles called chromosomes. See Figure 1.3. Abnormal changes (mutations) in genes cause normal cells to become cancer cells. Researchers are still trying to learn what causes genes to mutate and cause cancer.

Cancer cells don't behave like normal cells in three key ways. First, mutations in genes cause normal cells to grow more quickly and live longer. Normal cells grow and then divide to form new cells when needed. They also die when old or damaged as shown in Figure 1.4. In contrast, cancer cells make new cells that aren't needed and don't die quickly when old or damaged. Over time, breast cancer cells form a mass called the primary tumor.

The second way cancer cells differ from normal cells is that they can grow into surrounding tissues. If not treated, the primary tumor can extend beyond the walls of lobules or ducts into the stroma. Breast cancers that haven't grown into the stroma are called "noninvasive breast cancer." Breast cancers that have grown into the stroma, such as stages I and II, are called "invasive breast cancer."

Third, unlike normal cells, cancer cells can leave the breast and form tumors in other parts of the body. This process is called metastasis. In this process, cancer cells break away from the tumor and merge with blood or lymph. Then, the cancer cells travel in blood or lymph through vessels to other sites. The first site is your axillary lymph nodes. Common distant sites include your bones, lungs, brain, and liver. Once cancer cells are in other sites, they can form secondary tumors and may cause major health problems.

Figure 1.3
Genetic material in cells

Most human cells contain the "blueprint of life"—the plan by which our bodies are made and work. The plan is found inside of chromosomes, which are long strands of DNA that are tightly wrapped around proteins. Genes are small pieces of DNA that contain instructions for building new cells and controlling how cells behave. Humans have about 24,000 genes.

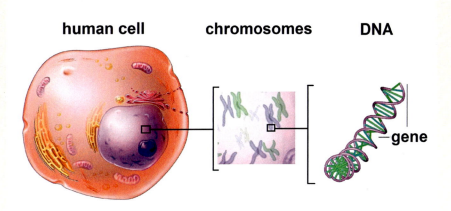

Illustration Copyright © 2016 Nucleus Medical Media, All rights reserved. www.nucleusinc.com

Figure 1.4
Normal cell growth vs. cancer cell growth

Normal cells increase in number when they are needed and die when old or damaged. In contrast, cancer cells quickly make new cells and live longer because of abnormal changes in genes.

Illustration Copyright © 2016 Nucleus Medical Media, All rights reserved. www.nucleusinc.com

Cancer stage

A cancer stage is a rating by your doctors of the extent of the cancer. It is used to plan which tests may be needed and which treatments are best for you. The AJCC (**A**merican **J**oint **C**ommittee on **C**ancer) staging system is used to stage breast cancer.

Rating of the cancer stage is often done twice. The first rating is based on tests before treatment and is called the clinical stage. Exactly how far the cancer has spread and how many axillary lymph nodes have cancer can't be known until after surgery. Thus, your doctors will rate the cancer again after surgery. This rating is called the pathologic stage.

Breast cancer has 5 stages ranging from 0 to IV. The focus of this book is on stages I and II. These breast cancers have grown into the stroma but not into the breast skin or chest wall. The cancer hasn't spread to distant sites. Clinical stages I and II are defined as:

Stage I
- Breast tumors are 2 cm (**c**enti**m**eters) or smaller in size and appear not to have spread to any lymph nodes.

Stage IIA
- Breast tumors are no larger than 2 cm or no breast tumor has been found. The cancer appears to have spread to a few axillary lymph nodes.
- Breast tumors are larger than 2 cm but no larger than 5 cm. There are no signs of cancer in any lymph nodes.

Stage IIB
- Breast tumors are larger than 2 cm but no larger than 5 cm. The cancer appears to have spread to a few axillary lymph nodes.
- Breast tumors are larger than 5 cm with no signs of cancer in any lymph nodes.

Treatment options

You will be making many choices about your treatment for breast cancer. One choice may be whether to join a clinical trial. Clinical trials assess how safe and helpful tests and treatments are. When found to be safe and helpful, tests and treatments from a clinical trial may become tomorrow's standard of care. Clinical trials are the treatment option that is preferred by NCCN experts. Ask your treatment team if there is an open clinical trial that you can join. You can also find clinical trials through the websites listed in Part 9.

If you will not be joining a trial, other options are briefly described next. As shown in **Figure 1.5**, treatment for stage I or II breast cancer has many parts. First, the cancer and your health will need to be assessed as discussed in *Part 2 Treatment planning*. Your treatment options will be based on test results.

This book focuses on cancer treatment, but supportive care is also important. Supportive care doesn't aim to treat cancer but aims to improve quality of life. It can address many needs. One example is treatment for physical and emotional symptoms. Supportive care can also help with treatment decisions as you may have more than one option. It can also help with coordination of care between health providers. Talk with your treatment team to plan the best supportive care for you.

1 Breast cancer basics | Treatment options

Figure 1.5 Common treatment path

Treatment for stages I and II breast cancer has many parts. As such, you will have many choices to face. Read Parts 2 through 8 to learn what your options are.

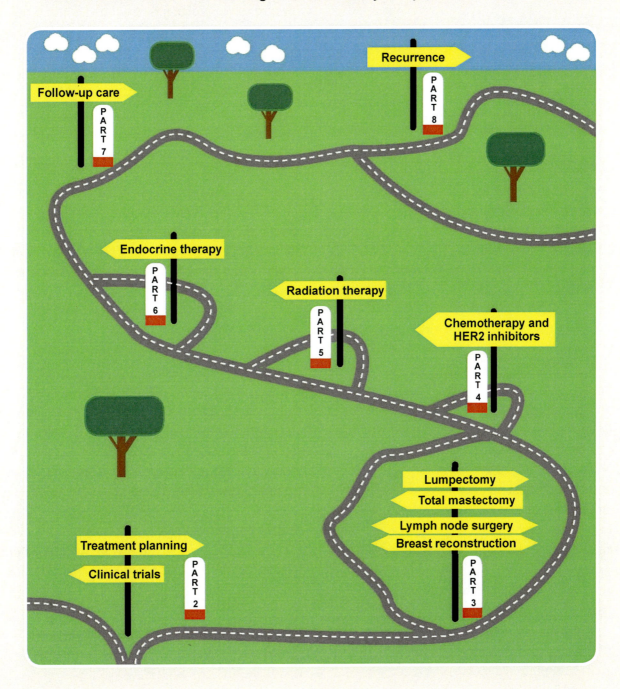

1 Breast cancer basics | Treatment options

Breast cancer surgery

Surgery to remove the cancer is a central part of treatment for stages I and II breast cancer. Cancer in the breast and any lymph nodes will be removed. However, other treatments will likely be used with surgery to treat the cancer.

Treatment for stages I and II breast cancer has many parts. As such, you will have many choices to face. Read Parts 2 through 8 to learn what your options are.

Lumpectomy and a total mastectomy are two types of breast surgery used for stages I and II breast cancer. A lumpectomy is a surgery that removes the tumor along with normal-looking tissue around its edge. The normal-looking tissue is called a surgical margin. Lumpectomy is a breast-conserving surgery because most of the normal breast tissue won't be removed. A total mastectomy is a surgery that removes the entire breast but not any chest muscle. *Part 3 Breast cancer surgery* presents which surgery is an option for you.

Surgery is often the first treatment for stages I & II breast cancer. It may not be the first treatment if you have a large breast tumor and want to have a lumpectomy. In this case, you may first receive cancer drugs to try to shrink the tumor. Use of cancer drugs for this purpose is called neoadjuvant (or preoperative) treatment.

At the time of the breast surgery, most women with stage I or II breast cancer will have some axillary lymph nodes removed. Lymph nodes will be removed by one or two methods. A sentinel lymph node biopsy is a surgery that finds and removes the first lymph nodes to which breast cancer spreads. It is also called a sentinel lymph node dissection. An axillary lymph node dissection removes more axillary lymph nodes than a sentinel lymph node biopsy. *Part 3 Breast cancer surgery* addresses which surgery is an option for you.

Breast reconstruction is a surgery that inserts breast implants or uses your body tissue to make a more normal-looking breast mound. Following the cancer surgery, or in some cases at the same time, you may want to have breast reconstruction. However, some women use external fake breasts or do nothing. Breast reconstruction is described in more detail in *Part 3 Breast cancer surgery*.

Chemotherapy and HER2 inhibitors

You may receive chemotherapy and HER2 (**h**uman **e**pidermal growth factor **r**eceptor **2**) inhibitors after surgery. These cancer drugs lower the chances of breast cancer returning. Treatment for this purpose is called adjuvant treatment. Chemotherapy, or "chemo," includes drugs that disrupt the life cycle of cancer cells. Thus, no new cells are made to replace dying cells. HER2 inhibitors stop certain signals that tell cancer cells to grow. *Part 4 Chemotherapy and HER2 inhibitors* addresses if these treatments are an option for you.

Radiation therapy

Radiation therapy uses high-energy rays to treat cancer. The rays damage the genes in cells. This either kills the cancer cells or stops new cancer cells from being made. If you will receive chemotherapy, radiation therapy is most often given afterward. Otherwise, radiation therapy follows surgery. *Part 5 Radiation therapy* addresses if radiation therapy is an option for you.

Endocrine therapy

Female hormones help some breast cancers grow. Endocrine therapy includes treatments that stop cancer growth caused by hormones. Endocrine therapy is sometimes called hormone therapy but is not the same as hormone replacement therapy. It is used as an adjuvant treatment and may be started during or after radiation therapy.

1 Breast cancer basics | Treatment options

There are 4 types of endocrine therapy. <u>Antiestrogens</u> are drugs that stop the effect of <u>estrogen</u> on cancer cell growth. <u>Aromatase inhibitors</u> are drugs that lower <u>estrogen</u> levels in the body. <u>Ovarian ablation</u> uses either surgery or <u>radiation therapy</u> to stop ovaries from making estrogen. <u>Ovarian suppression</u> is the use of drugs to stop the ovaries from making estrogen. *Part 6 Endocrine therapy* addresses if and what types of <u>endocrine therapy</u> are options for you.

Breast cancer recurrence

Testing to assess the outcomes of cancer treatment is part of follow-up care. Follow-up care is addressed in Part 7. Testing may show that the cancer has returned (<u>recurrence</u>). *Part 8 Breast cancer recurrence* addresses what types of treatment are options for you if the cancer returns.

1 Breast cancer basics | Review

Review

- Inside of women's breasts are lobules, ducts, and stroma. Lobules are structures that make breast milk. Ducts carry breast milk from the lobules to the nipple. Stroma is a soft tissue that surrounds the lobules and ducts.

- Breast cancer often starts in the lobules or ducts and then grows into the stroma.

- Breast cancer can spread outside the breast to vital organs through lymph or blood.

- Breast cancer that is stage I or II has grown into the stroma but not into the breast skin or chest wall. It has not spread to distant sites.

- Clinical trials are the treatment option that is preferred by NCCN experts. Other options involve surgery, chemotherapy, HER2 inhibitors, radiation therapy, endocrine therapy, follow-up care, and recurrence treatment. Parts 2 through 8 present what your options may be.

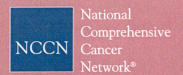

2
Treatment planning

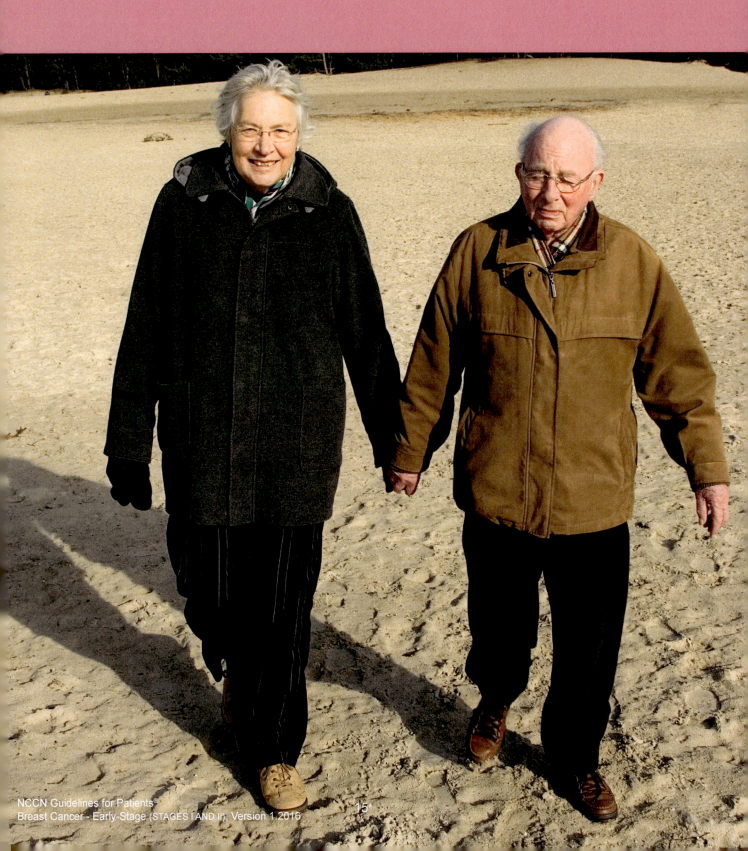

2 Treatment planning

16	Medical history
17	Physical exam
17	Blood tests
18	Imaging tests
21	Lymph node biopsy
22	Receptor tests
24	Genetic counseling
24	Fertility counseling
25	Distress screening
26	Review

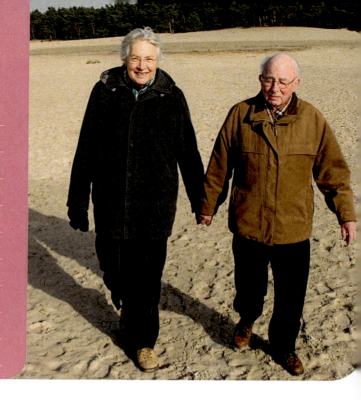

Doctors plan treatment with many sources of information. These sources include tests of your health and the cancer. Part 2 describes who should receive which tests before treatment. Some of these tests are repeated after treatment. Besides tests, Part 2 describes other types of care that are important to receive before cancer treatment.

Medical history

Your medical history includes any health events and medicines you've taken in your life. Your doctor will want to know about illnesses, breast biopsies, prior treatment with radiation, and if you are pregnant. It may help to make a list of old and new medications while at home to bring to your doctor's office.

Breast cancer and other health conditions can run in families. Thus, your doctor will ask about the medical history of your relatives. About 1 out of 10 breast cancers are due to abnormal genes that are passed down from a parent to a child. Such cancers are called hereditary breast cancer.

A medical history is one of the tests needed for treatment planning. **See Chart 2.1** for a complete list of care that is recommended prior to treatment. Some types of care are for anyone with stage I or II breast cancer while others may be useful for some women.

Physical exam

Doctors often perform a physical exam along with taking a medical history. A physical exam is a study of your body for signs of disease. During this exam, your doctor will listen to your lungs, heart, and gut.

Your doctor will also look at and feel parts of your body. This is done to see if organs are of normal size, are soft or hard, or cause pain when touched. A clinical breast exam involves your doctor touching your breasts and nearby lymph nodes. Your breasts may be felt while you sit or stand up as well as when you lie back. Some women feel uneasy having their breasts touched by their doctor. Keep in mind that this test provides important information and is quick.

Blood tests

Blood tests may be done to check for any health problems before starting treatment. For a blood test, a needle will be inserted into your vein to remove a sample of blood. The needle may bruise your skin and you may feel dizzy from the blood draw. Your blood sample will then be sent to a lab where a pathologist will test it.

Complete blood count

A CBC (complete blood count) measures the number of blood cells in a blood sample. It includes numbers of white blood cells, red blood cells, and platelets. Cancer and other health problems can cause low or high counts.

Chart 2.1 Health care before cancer treatment

Main tests and services	Other care based on signs and symptoms
• Medical history	• Complete blood count
• Physical exam	• Liver function tests
• Diagnostic bilateral mammogram	• Bone scan
• Ultrasound if needed	• Chest diagnostic CT
• Breast MRI is an option	• Abdominal ± pelvic diagnostic CT or MRI
• Pathology review	• Lymph node biopsy
• Hormone receptor test	
• HER2 test	
• Genetic counseling if hereditary breast cancer is likely	
• Fertility counseling if you can have babies	
• Distress screening	

2 Treatment planning | Imaging tests

Liver function tests

Your liver is an organ in the upper right side of your abdomen. It does many important jobs, such as remove toxins from your blood. Liver function tests assess for chemicals that are made or processed by the liver. Levels that are too high or low may signal that the cancer has spread to distant sites. One such chemical is ALP (alkaline phosphatase). High levels of ALP may mean that the cancer has spread to your liver or bones.

Imaging tests

Imaging tests make pictures (images) of the insides of your body. They can show which sites have cancer. This information helps your doctors stage the cancer.

Your treatment team will tell you how to prepare for these tests. You may need to stop taking some medicines and stop eating and drinking for a few hours before the scan. Tell your doctors if you get nervous when in small spaces. You may be given a sedative to help you relax.

Bilateral diagnostic mammogram

A mammogram is a picture of the insides of your breast. The pictures are made using x-rays. Mammograms that are used for breast cancer screening are often made from two x-rays of each breast. A computer combines the x-rays to make detailed pictures. See Figure 2.1 for more information.

Many women diagnosed with breast cancer have already had a bilateral diagnostic mammogram. If you haven't had this test, it is advised. A bilateral mammogram is a picture of each breast. Diagnostic mammograms are made with more x-rays from different angles than screening mammograms. By using more x-rays, the picture is clearer and can better show the size and number of tumors.

Ultrasound

Ultrasound is a test that uses sound waves to make pictures. For this test, you will need to lie down on a table. Next, a technician or doctor will hold the ultrasound probe on top of your breast. The probe may also be placed below your armpit to view your lymph nodes.

Breast MRI

If the mammography and ultrasound images are unclear, your doctors may want you to get a breast MRI (magnetic resonance imaging). This test uses a magnetic field and radio waves to make pictures of the insides of your breasts. Before the test, a contrast dye may be injected into your vein to make the pictures clearer. The dye may cause you to feel flushed or get hives. Rarely, serious allergic reactions occur. Tell your doctor if you have had bad reactions before.

For breast MRI, you must remove your top and bra and lie face down on a table. The table has padded openings for your breasts. In the openings, there are coils that help to make pictures. During breast MRI, the table moves slowly through the tunnel of the MRI machine.

Bone scan

A bone scan is recommended if you have bone pain or if ALP levels are high. Before the pictures are taken, a radiotracer will be injected into your vein. The most common radiotracer used for bone scans is technetium. You will need to wait about 3 hours for the radiotracer to enter your bones. A special camera is used to take pictures while you lie still on a table. It takes 45 to 60 minutes to complete the pictures. Areas of bone damage use more radiotracer than healthy bone and thus appear as bright spots. Bone damage can be caused by cancer as well as other health problems.

Figure 2.1 Mammogram

Mammograms are pictures of the insides of your breasts. They are often easy to get. Before the test, don't use deodorants, perfumes, powders, or lotions on your breasts and armpits or wash them off. These products can make the pictures unclear. You will also need to remove your top and bra.

In the exam room, a technician will tell you how to place your body next to the machine. Your breast will be placed onto a flat surface, called a plate. A second plate will be lowered onto your breast to flatten it. This may be painful but it gets the least fuzzy picture of your breast. Pictures will be taken from a camera that is attached to the two plates. Mammograms of both breasts take about 20 minutes to complete.

The pictures are either printed on film or saved on a computer. An expert in mammograms, called a radiologist, will view the pictures. He or she will report the test findings to your doctor.

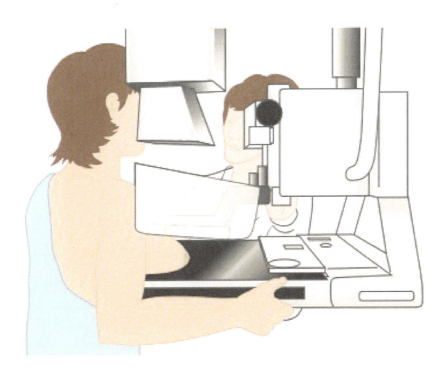

Diagram showing a woman having a mammogram by Cancer Research UK available at commons.wikimedia.org/wiki/File:Diagram_showing_a_woman_having_a_mammogram_CRUK_089.svg under a Creative Commons Attribution-Share Alike 4.0 International license.

2 Treatment planning | Imaging tests

Chest diagnostic CT

CT (computed tomography) takes many x-rays from different angles to make detailed pictures. You may get a CT scan of your chest if you have symptoms of lung disease. The CT scan can help show if the symptoms are caused by cancer or another health problem. Like a breast MRI, a contrast dye may be used. For the CT scan, you will need to lie face up on a table that moves through the machine.

Abdominal ± pelvic diagnostic CT or MRI

CT and MRI scans can be used to see the insides of your abdomen and pelvis. If you have symptoms in these areas, a scan can help show if the symptoms are caused by cancer or another health problem. Your doctors may also order a scan of these areas if the physical exam, ALP blood test, or liver function tests suggest a health problem.

Pathology report

A pathologist is a doctor who's an expert in testing cells to find diseases. This doctor confirms that cancer is present by viewing a sample of cells with a microscope. When cancer is found, he or she will do other tests to learn more about the cancer. All lab results are included in a pathology report that gets sent to your doctors.

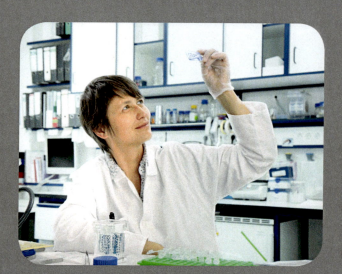

Some women get more than one pathology report. The first report may include the test results of a breast biopsy. Other pathology reports may include test results of breast tissue removed during surgical treatment. It's a good idea to ask for a copy of your pathology reports. Also ask your treatment team any questions about the test results. These reports are used to plan treatment.

Lymph node biopsy

Breast cancer may spread to lymph nodes. If your lymph nodes feel large upon physical exam, they may have cancer. Likewise, lymph nodes that don't look normal in imaging scans may have cancer.

No biopsy is needed before surgery if the physical exam and imaging results of your lymph nodes are normal. If cancer may be present, a sample of tissue must be removed and tested. The removal of tissue is called a biopsy. As shown in **Figure 2.2**, there are two types of lymph node biopsies used for stages I and II breast cancer. They are FNA (**f**ine-**n**eedle **a**spiration) and core needle biopsy.

Before a biopsy, you may be asked to stop eating, stop taking some medicines, or stop smoking. Local anesthesia may be given to reduce pain. An FNA removes a small group of cells from a node using a very thin needle and syringe. The needle used in a core needle biopsy is able to remove a solid tissue sample. For either biopsy, ultrasound may be used to guide the needle into the node. A biopsy is generally a safe test.

The biopsy samples will be sent to a lab and tested for cancer cells. Further testing of your lymph nodes may be done at the time of surgery even if the physical exam, imaging tests, and biopsy results are normal.

Figure 2.2 Lymph node biopsies

Breast cancer can spread to the lymph nodes by your armpit. Signs of cancer in lymph nodes can be found with a physical exam, imaging test, or both. If a test suggests there's cancer, a biopsy is needed. An FNA removes a small group of cells and a core needle biopsy removes a solid tissue sample.

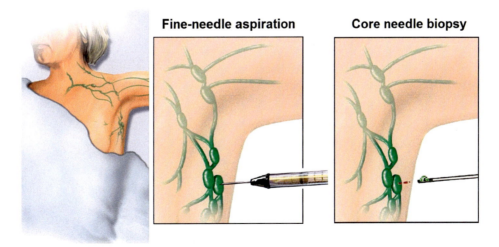

Illustration Copyright © 2016 Nucleus Medical Media, All rights reserved. www.nucleusinc.com

Receptor tests

Not all breast cancer cells are alike. Cancer cells can differ by the number or type of receptors they have. A receptor is a protein found in the membrane of cells or inside of cells. Substances bind to the receptors and cause changes within the cell. The two types of receptor tests important for treatment planning are:

Hormone receptor test

Estrogen and progesterone are hormones that are present in all women. Among some women with breast cancer, the cancer cells have receptors to which these hormones attach and cause the cells to grow in number. As shown in Figure 2.3, hormone receptors are inside of cells and enter the "control center," called the nucleus, after binding with estrogen. However, the growth of cancer cells with estrogen receptors is usually slower than cancer cells without these receptors.

Testing for estrogen receptors is important. There are drugs that can be used to stop hormones from causing cancer growth. IHC (immunohistochemistry) is the lab test used by pathologists for hormone receptors.

IHC involves applying a stain to cells then looking at them with a microscope. The stain shows how many cells have hormone receptors and the amount of hormone receptors in the cells. If at least 1 out of every 100 cancer cells stain positive, the cancer is called hormone receptor–positive. If fewer cancer cells stain positive for hormone receptors, the cancer is called hormone receptor–negative.

HER2 receptor test

In normal breast cells, there are two copies of the gene that makes HER2. As shown in Figure 2.3, HER2 is found within the membrane of cells. It extends from within the cell through the membrane to the outside of the cell.

When HER2 is activated, it causes breast cancer cells to grow and divide. Some breast cancers have cells with more than two copies of the gene that makes HER2. This causes too many HER2 receptors to be made. Other breast cancers have cells with only two HER2 gene copies but still too many HER2 receptors are made.

With too many HER2 receptors, breast cancer cells grow and divide fast. However, there are drugs to stop these cancer cells from growing. Due to high costs and the side effects of these drugs, it is very important to have tests that correctly show HER2 status. Like for hormone receptors, IHC is used to learn the amount of HER2 receptors. An IHC score of 3+ means that the cancer cells have many HER2 receptors. Another test of HER2 is ISH (in situ hybridization). ISH counts the number of copies of the HER2 gene. If the cancer cells have too many HER2 genes or receptors, the cancer is called HER2 positive.

Figure 2.3 Cell receptors in breast cancer

Hormone and HER2 receptors help breast cancer grow. Some women have a high amount of one or both types of receptors. It is important to test for these cell receptors so that the best cancer treatment is received.

a) Breast cancer that has too many cells with hormone receptors is called hormone receptor–positive.

b) Breast cancer that has too many HER2 receptors or genes is called HER2 positive.

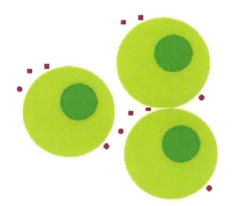
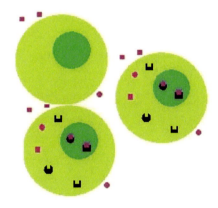

a. Hormone receptor–negative cancer   Hormone receptor–postive cancer

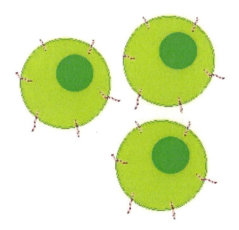
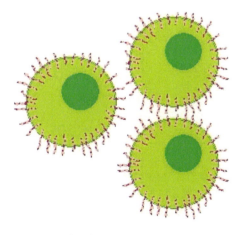

b. HER2-negative breast cancer   HER2-positive breast cancer

Genetic counseling

If you may have hereditary breast cancer, your doctor will refer you for genetic couseling. A genetic counselor is an expert in gene mutations that are related to disease. The counselor can tell you more about how likely you are to have hereditary breast cancer. He or she may suggest that you undergo genetic testing to look for gene mutations that increase your chances of developing breast cancer.

Hereditary breast cancer is most often caused by mutations in the *BRCA1* and *BRCA2* genes. Normal *BRCA* genes help to prevent tumor growth by fixing damaged cells and helping cells grow normally. Genetic testing can tell if you have a *BRCA* or another mutation. Your test results may be used to guide treatment planning.

Some abnormal changes in genes, called VUS (**v**ariants of **u**nknown **s**ignificance), are not fully understood by doctors. Your doctors may know of research that aims to learn more. If interested, ask your doctors about taking part in such research.

Fertility counseling

If you still have menstrual periods, your doctors will have important information to share with you. First, it is important that you not get pregnant during most cancer treatments. Cancer treatments may harm your baby. Your doctors can tell you which birth control methods are best to use while going through treatment.

Second, some breast cancer treatments may affect your ability to have babies in the future. If you want the choice of having babies after treatment or are unsure, tell your doctors. After treatment has ended, some women decide they want to have another baby.

If you still have menstrual periods, it may help to talk with a fertility specialist before you begin cancer treatment. A fertility specialist is an expert in helping women get pregnant. The fertility specialist can explain the ways to help you have a baby after treatment.

Distress screening

Distress is an unpleasant emotional state that may affect how you feel, think, and act. It can include feelings of unease, sadness, worry, anger, helplessness, guilt, and so forth. Everyone with cancer has some distress at some point in time. It is normal to feel sad, fearful, and helpless.

Feeling distressed may be a minor problem or it may be more serious. You may be so distressed that you can't do the things you used to do. Serious or not, it is important that your treatment team knows how you feel. They may ask you to complete a list of screening questions to assess how distressed you are.

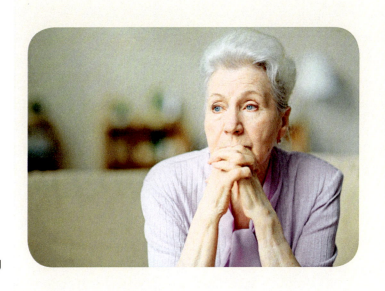

If needed, your treatment team can get you help. Help can include support groups, talk therapy, or medication. Some people also feel better by exercising, talking with loved ones, or relaxing. There may also be helpful community resources, such as support groups and wellness centers.

Review

- A medical history is a report of all health events in your lifetime. It will include questions about your family's health to help assess if you have hereditary breast cancer.

- Your doctor will examine your body for signs of disease. He or she will touch parts of your body, including your breasts, to see if anything feels abnormal.

- Imaging tests allow your doctor to see how far the cancer has spread without cutting into your body.

- An FNA or core needle biopsy of your lymph nodes may be done to test for cancer.

- Hormone and HER2 receptors can help breast cancer cells grow. Tests that assess the amount of these receptors are needed for treatment planning.

- Blood tests may be done to look for signs of cancer outside of your breast.

- Genetic counseling may help you decide whether to be tested for hereditary breast cancer.

- Fertility counseling may help you plan to have a baby when you're done with treatment.

- You should be screened for distress so you can receive help if needed.

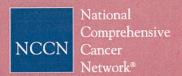

3 Breast cancer surgery

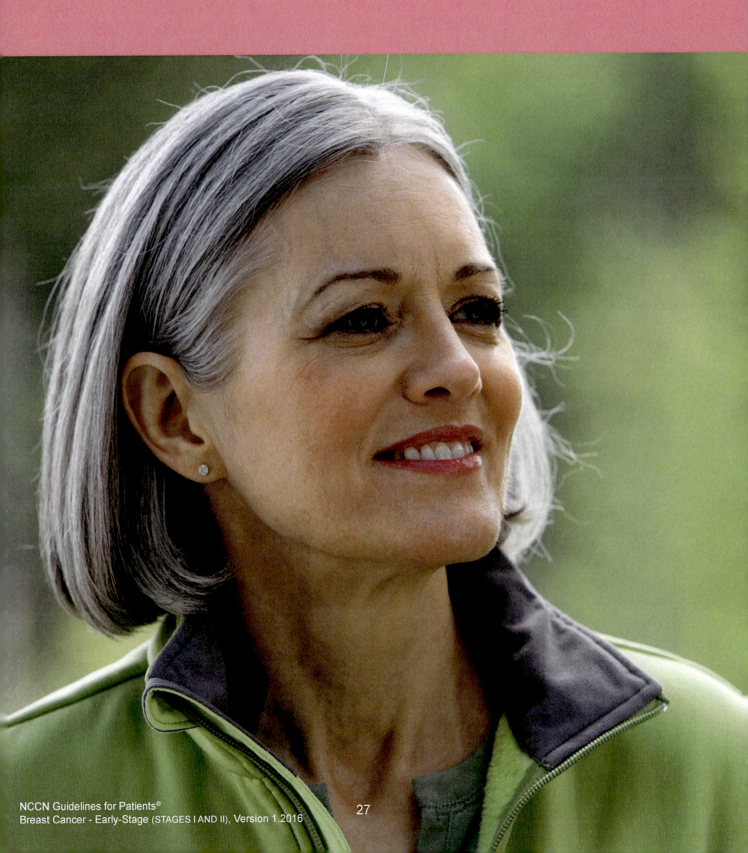

3 Breast cancer surgery

30　Breast tumor surgery
34　Lymph node surgery
38　Breast reconstruction
40　Review

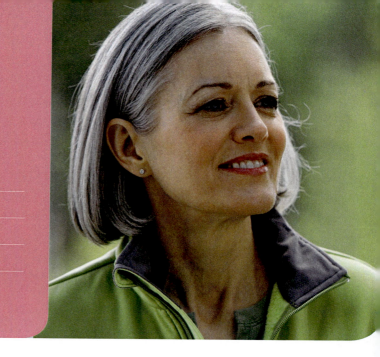

Surgery to remove cancer is a central part of treatment for stages I and II breast cancer. Part 3 explains which methods of removing the cancer may be options for you. It also provides some details on ways to rebuild breasts after cancer surgery.

Breast cancer that is stage I or II has not spread far if at all. As such, surgery to remove cancer in the breast and in any lymph nodes is a central part of treatment. In the section *Breast tumor surgery*, the two options for removing tumors from the breast are presented. Surgeries that remove lymph nodes are discussed in the section *Lymph node surgery*.

You may want to have your breasts re-shaped or re-made after the breast cancer is removed. The section *Breast reconstruction* contains information that may be of help.

Surgery is a "local treatment" since it treats cancer in a small part of your body. Most women will have another type of treatment after surgery to prevent the cancer from returning. Such treatments are presented in Parts 4 through 7.

My notes

Breast tumor surgery

Chart 3.1 Treatment options

Types of surgery	Deciding factors
Lumpectomy followed by radiation therapy (AKA breast-conserving therapy) is an option if *all* of these factors describe you	• Haven't had radiation close to where the cancer is, • Can have all cancer removed through one cut, • Have no health conditions that might cause problems, • Don't have a genetic risk for breast cancer, • Have cancer-free surgical margins, and • Your breast won't be too disfigured afterward.
Lumpectomy followed by radiation therapy (AKA breast-conserving therapy) may be an option if *any* of these factors describe you	• Have had prior radiation close to where the cancer is, • Have a breast tumor larger than 5 cm, • Are pregnant, • Have a connective tissue disease that affects your skin, • Have a genetic risk for breast cancer, or • Have a surgical margin with a limited area of cancer.
Total mastectomy is an option if *all* of these factors describe you	• Are unable or refuse to have an lumpectomy, and • Are healthy enough for surgery

Chart 3.1 lists deciding factors so you can know which breast surgery is an option for you. As shown in Figure 3.1, there are two types of breast surgery for stages I and II breast cancer. They are lumpectomy and total mastectomy. Other treatments may be used with breast surgery to rid your body of cancer.

Lumpectomy

A lumpectomy followed by radiation therapy is called breast-conserving therapy. It is an option for many but not all women with stage I or II breast cancer. The goal of a lumpectomy is to remove all the cancer in the breast while sparing healthy breast tissue. The deciding factors listed in the chart exclude women for

3 Breast cancer surgery | Breast tumor surgery

Figure 3.1 Breast tumor surgeries

Lumpectomy and mastectomy are two surgeries that remove cancer in the breast. Your treatment team will tell you how to prepare for and what to expect from surgery. Briefly, you will be asked to stop eating, drinking, and taking some medicines for a short period of time before the surgery. If you smoke, it is important to stop.

Lumpectomy
A lumpectomy removes the tumor along with a surgical margin. Pain is prevented with either local or general anesthesia. Often, breast tissue is removed through a C-shaped cut. A lumpectomy is finished within 15 to 40 minutes. A lumpectomy will leave a small scar and may cause some pain and swelling for about a week. It may also cause a dent in your breast that can be fixed with breast reconstruction.

Mastectomy
A total mastectomy removes the entire breast but not any chest muscle. Pain is prevented with general anesthesia. Often, an oval-shaped cut is first made around the nipple. Next, the breast tissue will be detached from the skin and muscle and then removed. A total mastectomy is finished within 1 to 2 hours. A total mastectomy will leave a large scar and cause pain and swelling. You may also have stiffness, severe tiredness despite sleeping (fatigue), and uncomfortable crawly sensations as your nerves heal.

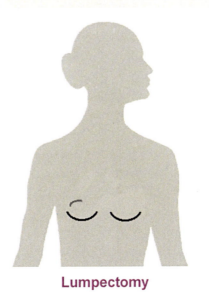
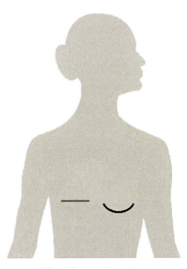

Lumpectomy   **Total mastectomy**

whom breast-conserving therapy would be unlikely to fully treat the cancer in the breast.

Tissue from a lumpectomy will be tested by a pathologist for cancer cells at or near the surgical margin. You also may be given another mammogram to look for any cancer that wasn't removed. If it appears that cancer remains in your breast, more surgery is needed. The second surgery is often another lumpectomy but sometimes a mastectomy is needed.

Neoadjuvant treatment

You may be able to have breast-conserving therapy even if you have a large stage II breast tumor. In this case, a breast tumor is large if it is bigger than 2 cm. Your doctors may decide that you can receive neoadjuvant (or preoperative) treatment to shrink the tumor.

If neoadjuvant treatment is planned, a core needle biopsy of the breast tumor is advised. A biopsy can confirm if there's cancer and what type. Your doctors will also assess for cancer in your axillary lymph nodes. Imaging tests and a biopsy of your lymph nodes may be done as described in Part 2.

Neoadjuvant treatment can cause the cancer to shrink a lot. Thus, the tumor sites in your breast and lymph nodes should be marked with small clips. Imaging tests, such as a mammogram or ultrasound, should be used to help place the clips. The clips will help your surgeon to find the tumor sites and remove tissue after neoadjuvant treatment.

Chemotherapy is the class of drugs most often used to shrink large breast tumors before surgery. Chemotherapy is discussed in Part 4. Endocrine therapy alone may be used for neoadjuvant treatment but only for some women with hormone receptor–positive cancer. Endocrine therapy is discussed in Part 6.

If you have HER2-positive breast cancer, you should be treated with chemotherapy and HER2 inhibitors for at least 9 weeks before surgery. For all neoadjuvant treatment, it is ideal that the full dose be given before surgery. If not completed, the remaining dose should be received after surgery.

During treatment you will be given tests to assess if the cancer is shrinking. Such tests include a physical exam and maybe imaging tests. If the cancer doesn't shrink much or grows, your doctor may give you a different type of chemotherapy. If the tumor shrinks enough, a lumpectomy can be done.

Total mastectomy

Some women with stage I or II breast cancer can't have or don't want a lumpectomy. A lumpectomy may not be an option because of your health, the tumor size, cancer in the surgical margins, and your chances of having another breast tumor.

You may refuse to have a lumpectomy. Some women refuse because of how they want their breast to look after treatment. Others refuse because they won't have to worry about the cancer returning in the removed breast.

If a lumpectomy isn't an option, a total mastectomy is advised. This surgery is also called a simple mastectomy. Your whole breast will be removed but not any chest muscle. Following the mastectomy, or in some cases at the same time as the mastectomy, you may want to have breast reconstruction. Breast reconstruction is described in more detail later in this chapter.

My notes

3 Breast cancer surgery | Lymph node surgery

Lymph node surgery

Chart 3.2 Treatment options

Type of surgery		Deciding factors
No lymph node surgery may be an option if *any* of these factors describe you	➡	• Have tubular or mucinous breast cancer, • Will have adjuvant treatment no matter what the results of lymph node surgery would be, • Are of older age, or • Have major health problems other than breast cancer.
Sentinel lymph node biopsy is an option if *any* of these factors describe you	➡	• Had a physical exam and imaging tests that showed no signs of cancer in your nodes, or • Had a FNA or core biopsy that found no cancer in nodes.

Axillary lymph node dissection is an option if *any* of these factors describe you	➡	• Had a physical exam or imaging test after neoadjuvant treatment that showed signs of cancer in your nodes,
		• Had an FNA or core needle biopsy that found cancer in your nodes and didn't have neoadjuvant treatment,
		• Had a sentinel biopsy that didn't find the sentinel node, or
		• Had a sentinel biopsy that found cancer in your lymph nodes plus one or more of the following:
		   ○ You have cancer in 3 or more nodes,
		   ○ You have a breast tumor larger than 5 cm,
		   ○ You will have a mastectomy,
		   ○ You won't have whole-breast radiation, or
		   ○ You will have neoadjuvant chemotherapy.

During the breast cancer surgery, axillary lymph nodes are often removed for cancer testing. By doing so, the cancer stage can be revised if needed. You are more likely to receive the best treatment when the cancer stage is correct.

Figure 3.2 shows the two types of lymph node surgeries. You may have one or both surgeries. It mainly depends on your results from the needle biopsy described in Part 2.

Chart 3.2 lists options for lymph node surgery. Some women may not need lymph node surgery because it likely wouldn't extend their life (survival). Such women include those with slow-growing cancers (tubular and mucinous breast cancers), set plans for adjuvant treatment, older in age, or those with major health problems other than breast cancer.

Sentinel lymph node biopsy

A sentinel lymph node biopsy is an option in two cases. It is an option if no signs of cancer were found in your lymph nodes by physical exam and imaging tests. It is also an option if no cancer was found in FNA or core needle biopsy samples. As explained next, some women who have a sentinel lymph node biopsy will need an axillary lymph node dissection.

Axillary lymph node dissection

An axillary lymph node dissection is needed in four cases. It is needed if after neoadjuvant treatment, a physical exam or imaging test suggests there's cancer in your nodes. Second, it is needed if cancer is found in FNA or core needle biopsy samples and you didn't have neoadjuvant treatment. Third, it is needed if the sentinel lymph node wasn't found with the sentinel lymph node biopsy. Last, it is needed if cancer was found in your sentinel nodes and there's more than a very small chance for the cancer to return.

Figure 3.2 Lymph node surgeries

To find sentinel lymph nodes, a radioactive tracer, blue dye, or both will be injected into your breast. The tracer and dye will drain into lymph vessels within your breast and then travel to the breast's lymph nodes. Often, there is more than one sentinel node. After the dye marks your sentinel node(s), it and likely some other nearby nodes will be removed through a second cut near the breast.

An axillary lymph node dissection removes at least 10 lymph nodes from Level I and II areas. Level I lymph nodes lie below the armpit. Level II lymph nodes are in the armpit. If cancer is found in Level II lymph nodes, nodes from Level III will be removed. Level III lymph nodes are below the collarbone.

Side effects are more common and can be more complicated with axillary lymph node dissection. Lymphedema is the most serious of these side effects. Lymphedema is swelling due to buildup of lymph and may not go away. Most women find lymphedema bothersome but not disabling. There is no way to know who will have it or when it will occur. Ask your treatment team for a full list of side effects caused by lymph node surgery.

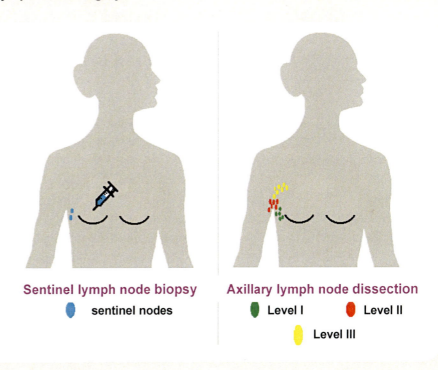

Breast reconstruction

Some women choose to have breast reconstruction after a lumpectomy or mastectomy. Options for breast reconstruction are described next. Talk with your doctor about these options.

Reconstruction following lumpectomy

If you will have a lumpectomy, your breast can be re-shaped using volume displacement. Volume displacement is the shifting of the remaining breast tissue so as to fill the hole left by the lumpectomy. Shifting of the breast tissue is often done by the cancer surgeon right after the lumpectomy.

A larger piece of breast tissue is removed during lumpectomy for volume displacement. Despite a larger piece, the natural look of your breast will be kept. Besides, having a larger piece removed will likely reduce your chances of cancer returning in that breast.

You may not like the results of the volume displacement. In this case, breast revision surgery may help. Breast revision surgery is done by a plastic surgeon. Other options include a second volume displacement, or you may want to get breast implants or flaps, which are described next.

Reconstruction following mastectomy

You can have reconstruction at any time if you have a total mastectomy. Reconstruction at the same time as the cancer surgery is called immediate reconstruction. Delayed reconstruction can occur months or years after the cancer surgery. Breast reconstruction following a mastectomy is done by a plastic surgeon.

To enhance your breast reconstruction, you may be able to have a skin-sparing mastectomy. This surgery usually removes only the nipple, areola, and skin near the biopsy site. As a result, the size of the mastectomy scar will be smaller and your breast will have a more natural shape. Skin-sparing mastectomy that spares the nipple and areola can be done for some women. Ask your surgeon if this is an option for you.

There is more than one way to reconstruct breasts and nipples after a mastectomy. All reconstruction is generally safe, but with any surgery, there are risks. Ask your treatment team for a complete list of side effects. The ways to reconstruct breasts and nipples are:

Implants

Breasts can be reconstructed using breast implants. Breast implants are small bags filled with salt water, silicone gel, or both that are placed under the breast skin and muscle. Implants have a small risk of breaking and leaking. A balloon-like device, called an expander, may first be placed under your muscle or skin and inflated to stretch out your muscle and skin. Every few weeks for two to three months, the expander will be enlarged until the implant will fit in place. You may feel pain from the expander stretching your skin and muscle. Some women will also have pain from the implant, scar tissue, or tissue death (necrosis).

Flaps

Another type of breast reconstruction uses tissue from your body, known as "flaps." Tissue is taken from the belly area, butt, or from under the shoulder blade to form breasts. See Figure 3.3. Some flaps are completely removed from your body and then sewn in place. Other flaps stay attached and then are slid over to the breast area and are sewn into place. Women who have high blood sugar (diabetes) or who smoke are more likely to have problems with flaps. Some risks of flaps are tissue death, lumps from death of fat, and muscle weakness that may cause organs to extend through (hernia).

3 Breast cancer surgery | Breast reconstruction

Implants and flaps

Some breasts are reconstructed with both implants and flaps. Using both types may give the reconstructed breast more volume and help match its shape to the other breast. However, for any reconstruction, you may need surgery on your real breast so that the two breasts match in size and shape.

Nipple replacement

Like your breast, you can have your nipple remade, use a fake nipple, or do nothing. The plastic surgeon can recreate a nipple mound with the surrounding tissues or, sometimes, tissue can be moved from other parts of your body. These other parts include your thigh, other nipple, or female parts between your legs (vulva). You may lose feeling in your real nipple if tissue is removed. Tissue used from other areas of your body to make a nipple can be darkened in color with a tattoo.

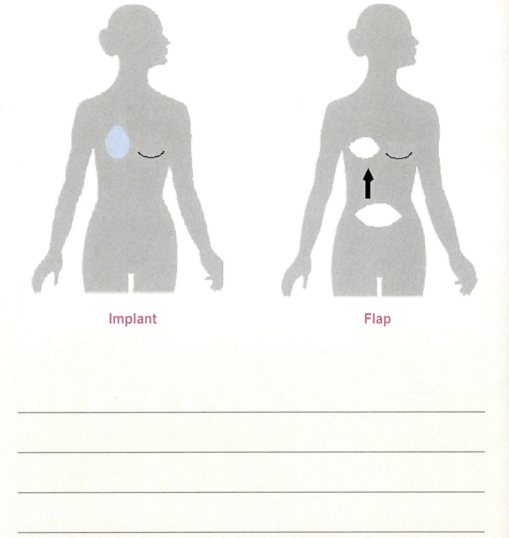

Figure 3.3 Breast reconstruction

Breast implants and flaps are the two main methods used for breast reconstruction following mastectomy. Implants are small bags filled with salt water, silicone gel, or both that are placed under your breast skin and muscle. Flaps are tissue taken from your belly area, butt, or from under your shoulder blade to form breasts.

Implant   Flap

3 Breast cancer surgery | Review

Review

- Lumpectomy and total mastectomy are the two breast tumor surgeries used for stages I and II breast cancer.

- Lumpectomy with radiation therapy is called breast-conserving therapy.

- Some women with a large breast tumor may be able to have breast-conserving therapy after receiving neoadjuvant treatment.

- Sentinel lymph node dissection removes the lymph nodes to which lymph first travels after leaving the breast.

- Axillary lymph node dissection removes sentinel lymph nodes and other lymph nodes around the armpit.

- Volume displacement is the shifting of the remaining breast tissue so as to fill the hole left by the lumpectomy.

- Breast reconstruction after mastectomy is done with breast implants, flaps, or both.

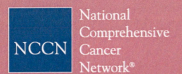

4
Chemotherapy and HER2 inhibitors

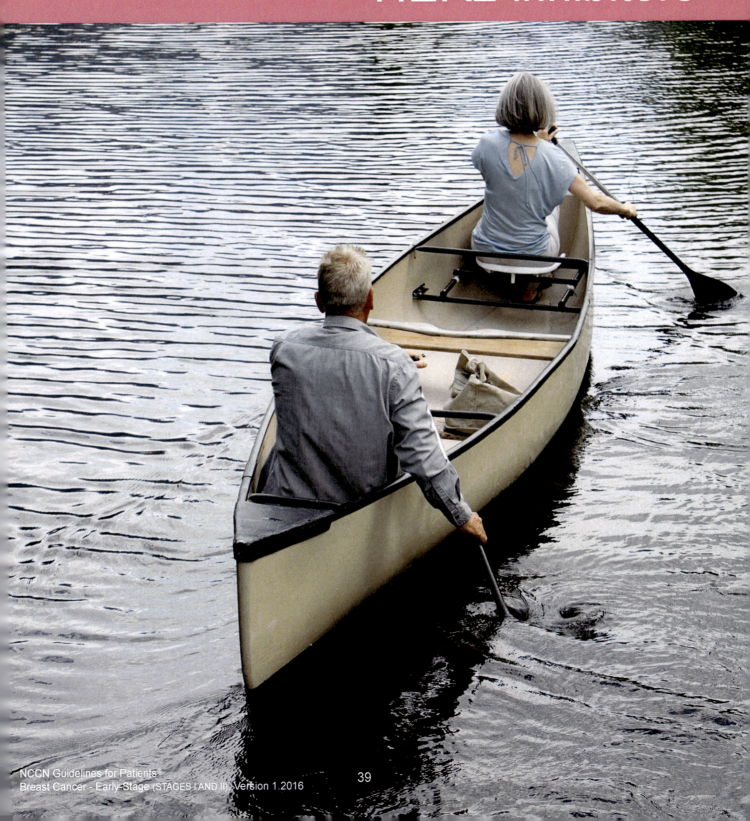

4 Chemotherapy and HER2 inhibitors

40 Overview
44 Treatment options
    44 HER-2 negative cancer
    46 HER-2 positive cancer
48 What to expect
50 Regimens
    50 HER-2 negative cancer
    52 HER-2 positive cancer
54 Review

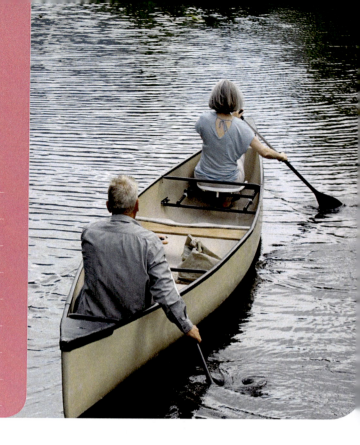

Some women with stage I or II breast cancer will receive chemotherapy with or without HER2 inhibitors. Part 4 explains who needs chemotherapy after surgery. It also presents some details on what to expect during chemotherapy and which drugs are used for stages I and II breast cancer.

Overview

Chemotherapy

Chemotherapy, or "chemo," is often given after surgery. It is given to lower the chances of breast cancer returning outside the breast. The chances of the cancer returning differ among women. Doctors predict the return of cancer based on features of the cancer and research results.

As explained in Part 3, chemotherapy is the first cancer treatment for some women with larger breast tumors. It is given to shrink the cancer. If the cancer shrinks enough, surgery may be an option.

Chemotherapy includes drugs that disrupt the life cycle of cancer cells. Some chemotherapy drugs kill cancer cells by damaging their DNA or by disrupting the making of DNA. Other drugs interfere with cell parts that are needed for making new cells. Thus, no new cells are made to replace dying cells.

4 Chemotherapy and HER2 inhibitors | Overview

As shown in Figure 4.1, some chemotherapy drugs work when cells are in an active growth phase. During the active growth phase, cells grow and divide to form a new cell. Chemotherapy drugs that disrupt the growth phase work well for cancer cells that are growing and dividing quickly. Other chemotherapy drugs work whether cells are in a growth or resting phase. Chemotherapy can kill both cancer and normal cells. Do not receive chemotherapy if you are in the first three months of pregnancy.

Figure 4.1 Cell phases

A cell goes through many changes to divide into two cells. Science has grouped these changes into 7 main phases. There may be another phase of rest, too. Some chemotherapy drugs work in any phase. Other chemotherapy drugs work in one or two growth phases.

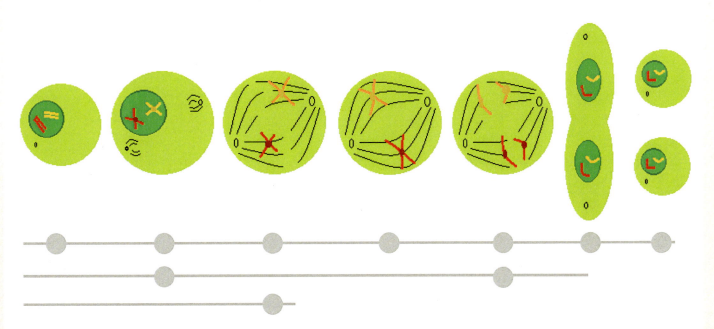

Chemotherapy may work in some or all phases of cell division

4 Chemotherapy and HER2 inhibitors | Overview

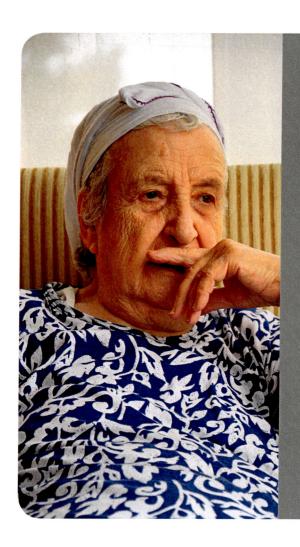

Chemotherapy after age 70?

The use of chemotherapy for women older than age of 70 has been questioned. You may not be given chemotherapy if you are older than 70 years for the following reasons. First, there is little research on older women to help inform treatment decisions. Second, chemotherapy may not be that helpful because the return of breast cancer can take a long time in older women. Thus, the odds that chemotherapy will stop a life-threatening recurrence are small. Third, some women have reactions to chemotherapy that threaten their health. Last, you may have health problems other than cancer that are more serious.

HER2 inhibitors

HER2 inhibitors are only used for HER2-positive breast cancer. They are monoclonal antibodies as explained in Figure 4.2. The HER2 inhibitors used for HER2-positive breast cancer are trastuzumab and sometimes pertuzumab. Trastuzumab is sold as Herceptin®, and pertuzumab as Perjeta®. Trastuzumab is always used with chemotherapy. Pertuzumab may be added if the breast cancer is stage II.

Figure 4.2 HER2 inhibitors

Antibodies are Y-shaped proteins that are made by your body to help fight illness. Monoclonal antibodies are human-made antibodies that attach to certain proteins on the outside of cancer cells. HER2 inhibitors are monoclonal antibodies, which are a type of targeted therapy.

Trastuzumab was the first HER2 inhibitor approved by the U.S. FDA in 1998 to treat HER2-positive breast cancer. Pertuzumab was approved in 2012. They attach to different parts of HER2. Thus, they stop growth signals from HER2 in different ways. Both of them also mark breast cancer cells for destruction by your body's disease-fighting (immune) system.

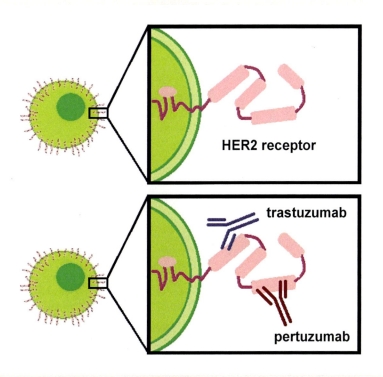

Treatment options: HER-2 negative cancer

Chart 4.1 Hormone receptor-negative (triple-negative breast cancer)

Size of breast tumor	Size of lymph node tumors	Do I need chemotherapy?
0.5 cm or smaller	No tumors	Unlikely
	Tiny (≤2.0 mm) tumors	Consider chemotherapy
0.51 to 1.0 cm	None or tiny (≤2.0 mm) tumors	Consider chemotherapy
Larger than 1.0 cm	Any size	Yes

Chart 4.2 Hormone receptor-positive

Size of breast tumor	Size of lymph node tumors	RT-PCR score	Do I need chemotherapy?
0.5 cm or smaller	No tumors	–	Unlikely
	Tiny (≤2.0 mm) tumors	–	Consider chemotherapy
0.51 or larger	None or tiny (≤2.0 mm) tumors	Not done	Consider chemotherapy
		<18	Unlikely
		18–30	Consider chemotherapy
		≥31	Yes
Any size	Larger than 2.0 mm	–	Yes

4 Chemotherapy and HER2 inhibitors | Treatment options: HER-2 negative cancer

There is more than one subtype of breast cancer. Receiving chemotherapy is partly based on the subtype. Chemotherapy is less often used to treat rare subtypes that are not likely to spread beyond the breast.

Tubular and mucinous breast cancers are rare subtypes of invasive ductal carcinoma. Tubular breast cancer is so named because the cancer cells look like tubes. Mucinous (or colloid) breast cancer is so named because there's a lot of mucus around the cancer cells. The chances are low that either subtype will spread outside the breast. Thus, chemotherapy is often not used.

Other subtypes of breast cancer have higher chances of spreading outside the breast. However, the chances for spreading are still low for most of these subtypes. Higher-risk subtypes include most forms of invasive ductal carcinoma as well as invasive lobular, metaplastic, and mixed carcinomas. Metaplastic carcinoma is breast cancer that changed from one cell type to another. Mixed carcinoma is breast cancer that has more than one cell type. Chemotherapy for these subtypes is discussed next.

Chart 4.1 shows when chemotherapy is advised for HER2-negative, hormone receptor–negative breast cancer. These cancers are called "triple-negative." Chemotherapy is also based on tumor size.

Chemotherapy isn't usually given if a breast tumor is 0.5 cm or smaller and hasn't spread. This is because the results of local treatment alone are often very good. In contrast, chemotherapy is advised if a breast tumor is 1.0 cm or larger. For all other tumors, your doctor may want you to have chemotherapy to lower the chances of the cancer returning.

Chart 4.2 shows when chemotherapy is advised for HER2-negative, hormone receptor–positive breast cancers. Chemotherapy is also based on tumor size. Chemotherapy isn't usually given if a breast tumor is 0.5 cm or smaller and hasn't spread. This is because the results of local treatment alone are often very good.

The 21-gene RT-PCR test looks at the activity of 21 genes to assess how likely it is that the cancer would return after local treatment. It is used to advise chemotherapy for breast cancers that are 0.51 cm and larger with no or little cancer growth in the axillary lymph nodes. Test scores range from 0 to 100. Chemotherapy should be considered if the test isn't done. A score below 18 means you can safely skip chemotherapy. A score of 18 to 30 means chemotherapy may be helpful. Scores of 31 and higher suggest that chemotherapy would help stop the return of breast cancer.

Chemotherapy is advised if at least one lymph node tumor is larger than 2 mm. However, some research supports the use of 21-gene RT-PCR to advise chemotherapy for women with cancer in 1 to 3 axillary lymph nodes. More research is still needed.

Treatment options: HER-2 positive cancer

Chart 4.3 Any hormone status

Size of breast tumor	Size of lymph node tumors	Do I need chemotherapy?
1.0 cm or smaller	None or tiny (≤2.0 mm) tumors	Consider chemotherapy with HER2 inhibitor(s)
Larger than 1.0 cm	None or tiny (≤2.0 mm) tumors	Yes, with HER2 inhibitor(s)
Any size	Larger than 2.0 mm	Yes, with HER2 inhibitor(s)

4 Chemotherapy and HER2 inhibitors | Treatment options: HER-2 positive cancer

Chart 4.3 shows when chemotherapy with HER2 inhibitor(s) is advised for HER2-positive breast cancers with any hormone status. Treatment is also based on tumor size. Your doctor may want you to have chemotherapy with HER2 inhibitor(s) if the breast tumor is 1 cm or smaller and there's none or little cancer growth in the axillary lymph nodes. Chemotherapy may help lower the chances of the cancer returning. Chemotherapy with HER2 inhibitor(s) is advised for breast tumors that are 1.0 cm or larger. Likewise, it is advised when at least one lymph node tumor is larger than 2 mm.

What to expect

Before chemotherapy, your doctor may ask you to stop taking some of your medicines, vitamins, or both. Some of these treatments can cause chemotherapy to not work as well or may cause health problems while on chemotherapy. Your doctor may ask you to eat a healthy diet and drink lots of fluids. If you smoke, it's important that you stop.

Chemotherapy drugs differ in the way they work, so often more than one drug is used. A combination regimen is the use of two or more chemotherapy drugs.

All chemotherapy drugs for stages I and II breast cancer are liquids that are injected into a vein. Only cyclophosphamide is made in pill form, too. The injection may be one fast shot of drugs into a vein or may be a slow drip called an infusion. Chemotherapy can also be given through a needle surgically placed in the chest or the arm. Trastuzumab and pertuzumab are given by infusion.

Chemotherapy is given in cycles of treatment days followed by days of rest. Giving chemotherapy in cycles gives your body a chance to recover after receiving chemotherapy. The cycles vary in length depending on which drugs are used.

You will need to go to a chemotherapy center to receive the drugs. How long your visit will be depends on what drugs you will get. It can take a few minutes or a few hours to finish a dose of chemotherapy. It takes about 90 minutes to get the first dose of trastuzumab and about 30 minutes for later doses. For pertuzumab, it takes about 60 minutes to get the first dose and about 30 to 60 minutes for later doses.

During chemotherapy cycles, you may be given other drugs to help you feel your best. You may be given drugs to fight nausea and vomiting. You may also

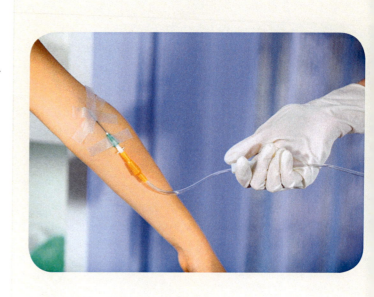

receive an injection under your skin the day after chemotherapy to increase the number of white blood cells to normal levels. Some people give themselves the injection while others return to the clinic for it. Blood, heart, and other tests may be given to check your health.

Side effects

The reactions to chemotherapy and HER2 inhibitors differ among women. Some women have many side effects. Other women have few. Some side effects can be very serious while others can be unpleasant but not serious.

Side effects of chemotherapy depend on the drug type, amount taken, length of treatment, and the person. In general, side effects are caused by the death of fast-growing cells. These cells are found in the hair follicle, gut, mouth, and blood. Thus, common side effects of chemotherapy include low blood cell counts, not feeling hungry, nausea, vomiting, diarrhea, hair loss, and mouth sores.

Other side effects of chemotherapy may include anxiety, fatigue, and peripheral neuropathy. Peripheral

4 Chemotherapy and HER2 inhibitors | What to expect

neuropathy is numbness or tingling of nerves in the hands and feet. Some types of chemotherapy, such as anthracyclines, can cause damage to the heart. Anthracyclines include doxorubicin and epirubicin.

Pre-menopausal women may start menopause early because of the chemotherapy drugs. Even if menstrual periods return after chemotherapy, you may still be unable to have babies. However, don't depend on chemotherapy for birth control. You may become pregnant while on chemotherapy, which can cause birth defects. If you had menstrual periods before chemotherapy, use birth control but not birth control made of hormones, such as "the pill." Talk to your doctors for more information.

You may have a mild flu-like response to the first dose of trastuzumab that includes fever, chills, headache, muscle aches, and nausea. This response is less common with the second and third doses. Other side effects may include damage to the heart and rarely to the lungs.

Common side effects of pertuzumab are diarrhea, nausea, and feeling tired and weak. Less common side effects include skin rash, low white blood cell counts, and mouth sores. It is not yet clear if pertuzumab damages the heart, although similar drugs do.

Not all the side effects of chemotherapy and HER2 inhibitors are listed here. Please ask your treatment team for a complete list. If a side effect bothers you, tell your treatment team. There may be ways to help you feel better.

4 Chemotherapy and HER2 inhibitors | Regimens: HER-2 negative cancer

Regimens: HER-2 negative cancer

Chart 4.4 Preferred regimens*

Preferred Regimen	Schedule	Total time
Dose-dense AC	Four 14-day cycles	4 months
then paclitaxel	Four 14-day cycles	
Dose-dense AC	Four 14-day cycles	5 months
then paclitaxel	Twelve 7-day cycles	
TC	Four 21-day cycles	3 months

Abbreviations
AC = doxorubicin + cyclophosphamide
CEF = cyclophosphamide + epirubicin + fluorouracil
CMF = cyclophosphamide + methotrexate + fluorouracil
EC = epirubicin + cyclophosphamide
FAC = fluorouracil + doxorubicin + cyclophosphamide
FEC = fluorouracil + epirubicin + cyclophosphamide
TAC = docetaxel + doxorubicin + cyclophosphamide
TC = docetaxel + cyclophosphamide

*Preferred and other regimens are based on how well they work, side effects, and treatment schedules.

4 Chemotherapy and HER2 inhibitors | Regimens: HER-2 negative cancer

Chart 4.5 Other regimens*

Other Regimen	Schedule	Total time
Dose-dense AC	Four 14-day cycles	2 months
AC	Four 21-day cycles	3 months
CMF	Six 28-day cycles	6 months
AC	Four 21-day cycles	6 months
then docetaxel	Four 21-day cycles	
AC	Four 21-day cycles	6 months
then paclitaxel	Twelve 7-day cycles	
EC	Eight 21-day cycles	6 months
FAC	Six 21-day cycles	7 months
then paclitaxel	Twelve 7-day cycles	
FEC or CEF	Four 21-day cycles	5 months
then paclitaxel	Eight 7-day cycles	
FEC or CEF	Three 21-day cycles	4 months
then docetaxel	Three 21-day cycles	
TAC	Six 21-day cycles	4 months

*Preferred and other regimens are based on how well they work, side effects, and treatment schedules.

Regimens: HER2-positive cancer

Chart 4.6 Preferred regimens*

Preferred Regimen	Schedule	Total time
AC	Four 21-day cycles	
then paclitaxel	Twelve 7-day cycles	1 year and 3 months
with trastuzumab	Weekly during paclitaxel then every 7 or 21 days to complete 1 year	
AC	Four 21-day cycles	
then paclitaxel	Four 21-day cycles	
with pertuzumab	Weekly during paclitaxel	1 year and 3 months
and trastuzumab	Weekly during paclitaxel then every 21 days to complete 1 year	
Dose-dense AC	Four 14-day cycles	
then paclitaxel	Four 14-day cycles	1 year and 2 months
with trastuzumab	Weekly during paclitaxel then every 7 to 21 days to complete 1 year	
TCH	Six 21-day cycles with weekly trastuzumab, then trastuzumab every 21 days to complete 1 year	1 year
TCH + pertuzumab	Six 21-day cycles with weekly trastuzumab and pertuzumab then trastuzumab every 21 days to complete 1 year	1 year

Chart 4.7 Other regimens*

Other Regimen	Schedule	Total time
AC	Four 21-day cycles	
then docetaxel	Four 21-day cycles	1 year and 3 months
with trastuzumab	Weekly during docetaxel cycles then every 21 days to complete 1 year	*Continues on next page.*

Abbreviations: AC = doxorubicin + cyclophosphamide; FEC = fluorouracil + epirubicin + cyclophosphamide; TCH = docetaxel + carboplatin + trastuzumab

*Preferred and other regimens are based on how well they work, side effects, and treatment schedules.

4 Chemotherapy and HER2 inhibitors | Regimens: HER-2 positive cancer

Chart 4.7 Other regimens* *Continued from previous page.*

Other Regimen	Schedule	Total time
AC	Four 21-day cycles	1 year and 3 months
then docetaxel	Four 21-day cycles	
with pertuzumab	On day 1 during docetaxel cycles	
and trastuzumab	On day 1 during docetaxel cycles then every 21 days to complete 1 year	
Docetaxel + cyclophosphamide	Four 21-day cycles	1 year
with trastuzumab	Weekly during docetaxel cycles then every 21 days to complete 1 year	
FEC	Three 21-day cycles	1 year and 9 weeks
then docetaxel	Three 21-day cycles	
with pertuzumab	On day 1 during docetaxel cycles	
and trastuzumab	On day 1 during docetaxel cycles then every 21 days to complete 1 year	
FEC	Three 21-day cycles	1 year and 9 weeks
then paclitaxel	Three 21-day cycles	
with pertuzumab	On day 1 during paclitaxel cycles	
and trastuzumab	On day 1 during paclitaxel cycles then every 21 days to complete 1 year	
Paclitaxel	Twelve 7-day cycles	1 year
with trastuzumab	Weekly during paclitaxel then every 7 or 21 days to complete 1 year	
Neoadjuvant docetaxel	Four 21-day cycles	3 months
with trastuzumab and pertuzumab, and	On day 1 during docetaxel cycles	
Adjuvant FEC	Three 21-day cycles	1 year and 9 weeks
then trastuzumab	Every 21 days to complete 1 year	
Neoadjuvant paclitaxel	Four 21-day cycles	3 months
with trastuzumab and pertuzumab, and	On day 1 during docetaxel cycles	
Adjuvant FEC	Three 21-day cycles	1 year and 9 weeks
then trastuzumab	Every 21 days to complete 1 year	

*Preferred and other regimens are based on how well they work, side effects, and treatment schedules.

4 Chemotherapy and HER2 inhibitors | Review

Review

- Chemotherapy is given after surgery to lower the chances of breast cancer returning outside the breast.

- In some cases, chemotherapy may be given before surgery to help shrink the cancer before surgery.

- You may not need chemotherapy if the breast cancer is a tubular and mucinous subtype.

- The need for chemotherapy to treat other subtypes depends on multiple factors including the size of tumors.

- You should take a HER2 inhibitor with chemotherapy if the cancer is HER2-positive.

- Chemotherapy is almost always a liquid that is slowly injected into a vein by infusion. It is given in cycles of treatment days followed by days of rest.

- Chemotherapy and HER2 inhibitors can cause side effects. Ask your treatment team for a complete list.

- There are multiple chemotherapy regimens that can be used to treat breast cancer. Talk to your doctor about which ones are best for you.

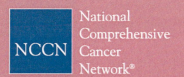

5 Radiation therapy

5 Radiation therapy

58 Treatment options
   58 After lumpectomy
   60 After mastectomy
62 What to expect
64 Review

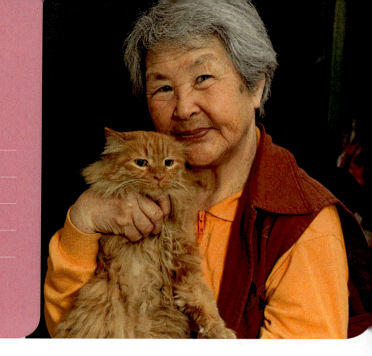

Many women with stage I or II breast cancer will receive radiation therapy. Part 5 explains who needs radiation therapy and which body sites should be treated. It also provides some details on what to expect during radiation therapy.

Radiation therapy is given to stop the return of cancer within the breast, nearby sites, or both. Doctors decide which sites need radiation based mainly on how many axillary lymph nodes have cancer. The more nodes with cancer the farther they think the cancer has spread.

Radiation therapy is usually given after chemotherapy is finished. It is okay to take HER2 inhibitors during radiation therapy. If you didn't have chemotherapy, radiation therapy follows surgery. If you are pregnant, don't start radiation until after your baby is born.

Radiation therapy uses high-energy rays to treat cancer. The rays damage the DNA in cells. This either kills the cancer cells or stops new cancer cells from being made. Radiation can also harm normal cells.

My notes

Treatment options after lumpectomy

Chart 5.1 Radiation guide

Results of lymph node surgery	Where do I need radiation?

No cancer in axillary nodes	• Whole breast with or without added boost to tumor site,
	• Part of the breast for some women, **or**
	• No radiation is needed if all of these factors describe you:
	  o You are 70 years old or older,
	  o The breast tumor was smaller than 2 cm,
	  o The cancer cells are hormone receptor–positive, and
	  o You will be taking endocrine therapy.

Cancer in 1 to 3 axillary nodes	• Whole breast with or without added boost to tumor site, **and** • Strongly consider treating supraclavicular and infraclavicular areas, internal mammary lymph nodes, and axillary areas at risk for cancer.
Cancer in 4 or more axillary nodes	• Whole breast with or without added boost to tumor site, • Supraclavicular and infraclavicular areas, • Internal mammary lymph nodes, **and** • Axillary areas at risk for cancer.

Chart 5.1 lists options for radiation therapy after having a lumpectomy. Options are based on how many axillary lymph nodes have cancer. Radiation to the breast is given only after cancer-free surgical margins have been removed. Possible radiation sites are shown in **Figure 5.1**.

Most women with cancer-free nodes receive radiation to the whole breast. This is called whole breast radiation. Toward the end of radiation, you may receive extra radiation called a boost if the cancer is likely to return after treatment.

Some women with cancer-free nodes receive partial breast irradiation. Partial breast irradiation is radiation given only to the lumpectomy site. More research is needed to know how well this treatment works.

If you're interested, it may be best to receive partial breast irradiation within a clinical trial. Outside of a clinical trial, partial breast irradiation is safest in treating breast cancer among women 1) who are 60 years of age or older; 2) with hormone receptor–positive ductal carcinoma that is confined to a small area with the breast; and 3) treated with surgery that had cancer-free surgical margins.

5 Radiation therapy | Treatment options after lumpectomy

Some women with cancer-free nodes are able to go without radiation. Such women include those older in age with small, hormone receptor–positive breast tumors who will be taking endocrine therapy. Endocrine therapy will likely stop the cancer from returning.

If the axillary lymph nodes weren't cancer-free, your whole breast should be treated. A boost may follow if the cancer is likely to return after treatment. The internal mammary lymph nodes and supraclavicular, infraclavicular, and axillary areas may be treated if 1 to 3 axillary nodes have cancer and should be treated if 4 or more nodes have cancer.

Figure 5.1 Radiation after lumpectomy

Most women will have radiation therapy after a lumpectomy. This combined treatment is called breast-conserving therapy. Most often, the whole breast is radiated. Other sites may be radiated if the axillary lymph nodes have cancer.

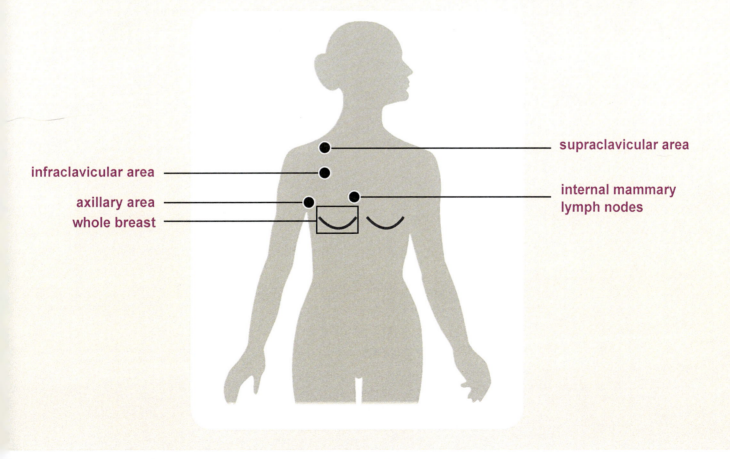

Treatment options after mastectomy

Chart 5.2 Radiation guide

Results of surgery	Where do I need radiation?
• No cancer in axillary lymph nodes, • Breast tumor is 5 cm or smaller, and • No cancer cells near edge of surgical margin that is 1 mm or larger	• No radiation therapy is needed.
• No cancer in axillary lymph nodes, • Breast tumor is 5 cm or smaller, and • No cancer cells near edge of surgical margin that is smaller than 1 mm	• Consider treating the chest wall.

• No cancer in axillary lymph nodes, and
• Breast tumor is larger than 5 cm or there are cancer cells at edge of surgical margin
	• Strongly consider treating the chest wall ± these sites:
	  o Axillary sites at risk for cancer,
	  o Supraclavicular and infraclavicular areas, and
	  o Internal mammary lymph nodes.

• Cancer in 1 to 3 axillary lymph nodes	• Strongly consider treating the chest wall + these sites:
	  o Axillary sites at risk for cancer,
	  o Supraclavicular and infraclavicular areas, and
	  o Internal mammary lymph nodes.

• Cancer in 4 or more axillary lymph nodes	• The chest wall, • Axillary sites at risk for cancer, • Supraclavicular and infraclavicular areas, and • Internal mammary lymph nodes.

5 Radiation therapy | Treatment options after mastectomy

Chart 5.2 lists options for radiation therapy after having a mastectomy. If your axillary lymph nodes are cancer-free, radiation therapy is advised based on the chances of the cancer returning after treatment. Breast cancer is more likely to return the larger a breast tumor is and the smaller a cancer-free surgical margin is. Despite cancer-free nodes, your doctor may advise radiation therapy if the surgical margin is smaller than 1 mm, the breast tumor is larger than 5 cm, or there's cancer in the surgical margin. Possible radiation sites are shown in Figure 5.2.

When cancer is found in 1 to 3 axillary lymph nodes, you may receive radiation therapy to multiple sites. These sites include the chest wall; supraclavicular, infraclavicular, and axillary areas; and the internal mammary lymph nodes.

If cancer is in 4 or more axillary lymph nodes, the breast cancer is upstaged to stage III. Radiation therapy is advised. Radiation sites include the chest wall; supraclavicular, infraclavicular, and axillary areas; and the internal mammary lymph nodes.

Figure 5.2 Radiation after mastectomy

Radiation therapy after mastectomy is based on how likely the cancer will return. The chest wall behind the removed breast may be radiated. Other sites include areas near the collarbone and armpit as well as lymph nodes along the breastbone.

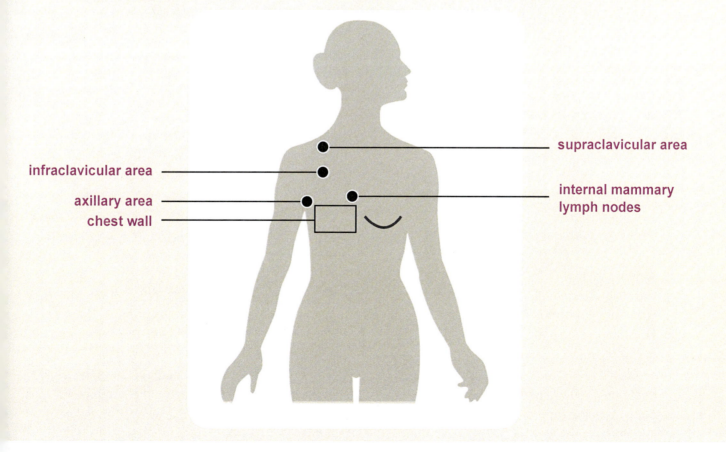

5 Radiation therapy | What to expect

What to expect

External radiation

The most common type of radiation therapy used for breast cancer is EBRT (external beam radiation therapy). This type of therapy uses a machine outside the body to deliver radiation. 3D machines deliver beams matched to the shape of the tumor. IMRT (intensity-modulated radiation therapy) uses small radiation beams of different strengths based on the thickness of the tissue.

A planning (simulation) session is needed before treatment. During simulation, pictures of the tumor site should be made with CT. Your doctors will use the pictures to decide the radiation dose and to shape the radiation beams. Beams are shaped with computer software and hardware added to the radiation machine. The beams are shaped so that normal tissue is spared. Radiation beams will be aimed at the tumor site with help from ink marks or tiny tattoos on your skin.

There are other methods that can be used to spare normal tissue. Moreover, there are ways to protect your heart if radiation will be given in that area. Ask your doctor what methods will be used for your treatment. Some methods are:

- Directing the beam not toward the heart,
- Lying face down during treatment,
- Holding your breath at times during treatment,
- Use of devices that keep you from moving during treatment,
- Radiation machines that give treatment only when the tumor is in the right spot, and
- Radiation machines that deliver very precise radiation beams.

During treatment, you will be alone while a technician operates the machine from a nearby room. He or she will be able to see, hear, and speak with you

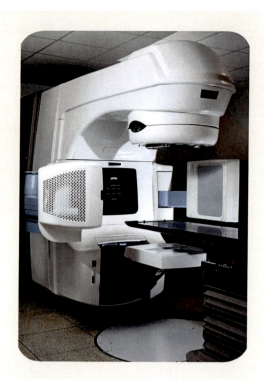

at all times. As treatment is given, you may hear noises. A session can take between 15 to 30 minutes. Radiation therapy is often given up to 5 days a week for 5 to 7 weeks but may be done quicker for some women.

Internal radiation

Some women receive a boost toward the end of their radiation therapy. The boost may be given with EBRT or by internal radiation. Internal radiation is also called brachytherapy. It involves placing radioactive seeds in the area where the tumor was. The seeds are placed using multiple small tubes (catheters) or one small catheter with a balloon at its end.

For multiple-catheter boost radiation, the seeds may remain in your body for minutes or days. If the seeds release a small dose of radiation, the catheters and seeds are left in your body for a few days. During this time, you must stay in the hospital. If the seeds release high doses of radiation, the seeds will remain in your body for 10 minutes. However, radiation is given twice a day for 5 days.

5 Radiation therapy | What to expect

Side effects

You may have side effects from radiation, although not everyone does. Often, the treated skin will look and feel as if it has been sunburned. It will likely become red and may also become dry, sore, and be painful when touched. Another common problem is extreme tiredness despite sleep (fatigue). Women sometimes have pain in their armpit or chest after radiation and rarely, heart and lung problems.

Not all the side effects of radiation have been listed here. Please ask your treatment team for a complete list of side effects. If a side effect bothers you, tell your treatment team. There may be ways to help you feel better.

Review

- The number of axillary lymph nodes is used to decide which sites need radiation therapy after lumpectomy. Most women receive at least whole breast radiation.

- The number of axillary lymph nodes and sometimes other factors are used to decide which sites need radiation therapy after mastectomy. Radiation is advised if cancer is present in four or more nodes.

- External beam radiation therapy is the most common type of radiation treatment for breast cancer.

- Radiation can cause your skin to feel sunburned and you to feel tired despite getting sleep.

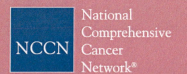

6
Endocrine therapy

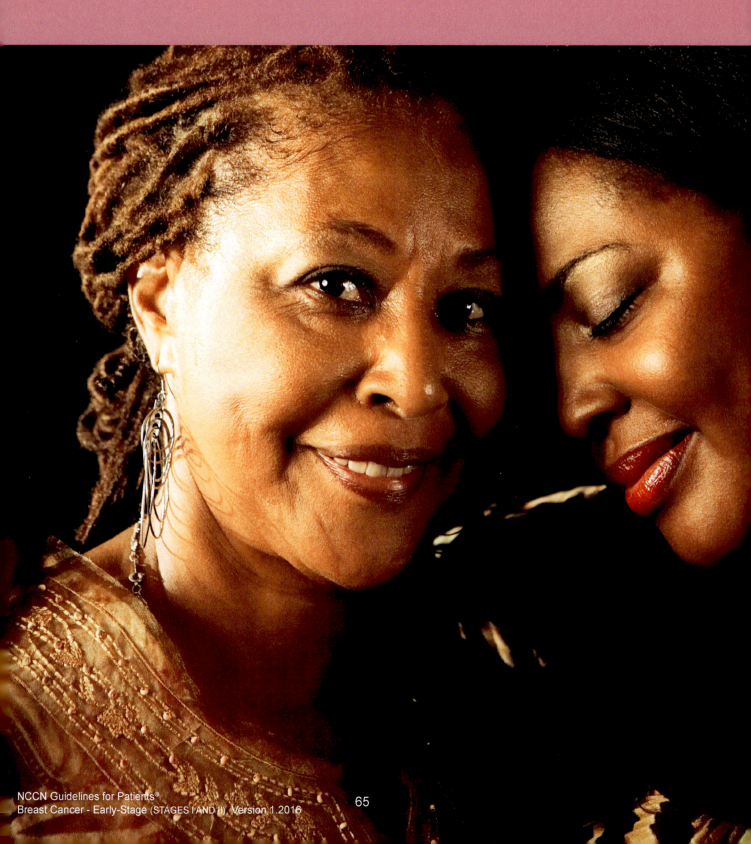

6 Endocrine therapy

68 Treatment options
70 What to expect
72 Regimens
74 Review

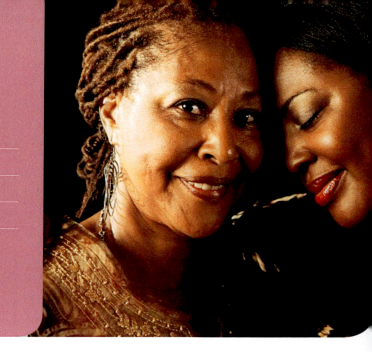

Many women with hormone receptor–positive breast cancer receive endocrine therapy. Part 6 explains who needs endocrine therapy and which types. It also provides some details on what to expect during endocrine therapy.

Estrogen and progesterone are hormones that cause some breast cancer cells to grow. Endocrine therapy stops the growth of cancer cells that is caused by hormones. It either lowers the amount or stops the effect of hormones in the body.

Endocrine therapy can be used to lower the chances of the cancer returning after surgery. It only works for women with hormone receptor–positive breast cancer. The chances of the cancer returning differ among women. Doctors predict the return of cancer based on features of the cancer and research results.

If you will receive chemotherapy, endocrine therapy should be started after chemotherapy is finished. It is okay to take HER2 inhibitors during endocrine therapy. Endocrine therapy can be started during or after radiation therapy. If you are pregnant, start endocrine therapy, if needed, after your baby is born.

My notes

6 Endocrine therapy | Treatment options

Treatment options

Chart 6.1 Endocrine therapy guide for hormone receptor-positive cancer

Size of breast tumor	Size of lymph node tumors	Do I need endocrine therapy?
0.5 cm or smaller	No tumors	Consider endocrine therapy
	Tiny (≤2.0 mm) tumors	Yes
Larger than .5 cm	None or tiny (≤2.0 mm) tumors	Yes
Any size	Larger than 2.0 mm	Yes

6 Endocrine therapy | Treatment options

As described in Part 4, there are rare subtypes of breast cancer that tend not to spread outside the breast. These rare, lower-risk subtypes include tubular and mucinous carcinomas. If the extent of a rare cancer is small, you may want to take endocrine therapy to prevent cancer in a breast that didn't have cancer. Endocrine therapy would also further reduce the small chance of cancer returning in the breast that was treated for cancer. Endocrine therapy is advised for lower-risk cancers if the breast tumor is 3 cm or larger or a tumor in a lymph node is larger than 2 mm.

Chart 6.1 shows when endocrine is advised for higher-risk subtypes that are hormone receptor–positive. Higher-risk subtypes include the more common breast cancers. Endocrine therapy is also based on tumor size.

Endocrine therapy is an option if a breast tumor is 0.5 cm or smaller and hasn't spread. The results of local treatment alone are often very good. In contrast, endocrine treatment is advised if a breast tumor is larger than 0.5 cm or lymph node tumors are present.

6 Endocrine therapy | What to expect

What to expect

There are four main types of endocrine therapy. Not all types will work for every woman. The types of treatment that may work for you depend on your menopausal status.

In general, menopause is the point in time when you won't have another menstrual period again. Breast cancer doctors also define menopause as when the ovaries aren't able to make high levels of estrogen. If you had your ovaries removed (oophorectomy) you are postmenopausal. If you had your uterus removed (hysterectomy), you may need blood tests to confirm your menopausal status. If you have these female organs but didn't have a menstrual period the year before cancer treatment, you are likely postmenopausal.

If you get menstrual periods, you are premenopausal. If you were premenopausal before starting chemotherapy, the absence of menstrual periods after chemotherapy doesn't mean you're postmenopausal. Your ovaries may still be working despite no menstrual periods or may start working again. To confirm your menopausal status, the amount of estrogen or FSH (follicle-stimulating hormone) in your blood needs to be tested.

Estrogen is mostly made by the ovaries and made in small amounts by the adrenal glands, liver, and body fat. Progesterone is also mostly made by the ovaries. The ovaries are the main source of estrogen and progesterone only in women who have menstrual periods (premenopausal). Endocrine therapy either blocks hormones from working or lowers hormone levels by targeting the main source.

Antiestrogens

Antiestrogens are drugs that stop the effect of estrogen on cancer cell growth. These drugs can be used among both premenopausal and postmenopausal women. Tamoxifen is an antiestrogen that is commonly used for stages I and II breast cancer.

As shown in **Figure 6.1**, tamoxifen treats breast cancer by attaching to the estrogen receptors and blocking estrogen from attaching. This type of antiestrogen is called a SERM (**s**elective **e**strogen **r**eceptor **m**odulator). It is a pill that is taken every day during the course of treatment.

Aromatase inhibitors

Aromatase inhibitors are drugs that lower estrogen levels in the body. These drugs work by blocking a protein that makes estrogen in postmenopausal women. They can't stop the ovaries in premenopausal women from making estrogen. For this reason, these drugs are only used among women after menopause caused by age or treatment. Three drugs in this category are: anastrozole (Arimidex®), letrozole (Femara®), and exemestane (Aromasin®). Each is a pill that is taken every day during the course of treatment.

Ovarian suppression

Ovarian suppression lowers the amount of estrogen in the body among premenopausal women. It is achieved with drugs called LHRH (**l**uteinizing **h**ormone-**r**eleasing **h**ormone) agonists. LHRH is a hormone in the brain that helps control the making of estrogen by the ovaries. LHRH agonists stop LHRH from being made, which stops the ovaries from making more estrogen. Goserelin (Zoladex®) and leuprolide (Eligard®, Lupron®) are LHRH agonists and are given as monthly injections under the skin.

Ovarian ablation

Ovarian ablation is the removal or destruction of the ovaries. This treatment stops the ovaries from making estrogen in premenopausal women. Surgery that removes both ovaries is called a bilateral oophorectomy. Radiation therapy to the ovaries

Figure 6.1 Antiestrogens

Antiestrogens are drugs that stop the effect of estrogen on cancer cell growth. Tamoxifen is an antiestrogen that is commonly used for stages I and II breast cancer. It blocks estrogen from attaching to its receptor and starting cell growth.

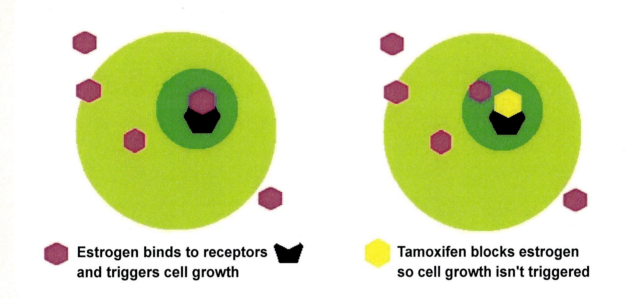

Estrogen binds to receptors and triggers cell growth

Tamoxifen blocks estrogen so cell growth isn't triggered

also stops the ovaries from making estrogen and progesterone, but isn't used often.

Side effects

For many women, endocrine therapy causes symptoms of menopause. Menopausal symptoms include hot flashes, vaginal discharge or dryness, sleep problems, weight gain, hair thinning, fatigue, and changes in mood. Which symptoms you will have may differ from other women.

Tamoxifen also has two rare but important side effects. They are cancer of the uterus and blood clots. For most women with breast cancer, the benefits of taking tamoxifen far outweigh the dangers.

Aromatase inhibitors don't cause cancer and very rarely cause blood clots. However, they can weaken your bones (osteoporosis) and cause bone fractures. Checking your bone health with regular bone mineral density tests can show bone weakness before fractures occur. Your doctor can order medicine to strengthen your bones if necessary. Aromatase inhibitors can also cause joint pain in some women.

Not all the side effects of endocrine therapy are listed here. Please ask your treatment team for a list of all common and rare side effects. If a side effect bothers you, tell your treatment team. There may be ways to help you feel better.

Regimens

Chart 6.2 Premenopausal women

Initial treatment	Extended treatment
• Tamoxifen for 5 years ± ovarian suppression or ablation	If still premenopausal: • Consider taking tamoxifen for another 5 years, or • Stop taking endocrine therapy If postmenopausal: • Take aromatase inhibitors for 5 years, or • Consider taking tamoxifen for another 5 years
• Aromatase inhibitor for 5 years + ovarian suppression or ablation	

Chart 6.3 Postmenopausal women

Initial, sequential, and extended treatment
• Aromatase inhibitor for 5 years
• Tamoxifen for 2–3 years followed by an aromatase inhibitor to complete 5 years of endocrine therapy
• Tamoxifen for 2–3 years followed by an aromatase inhibitor taken for up to 5 years
• Aromatase inhibitor for 2–3 years followed by tamoxifen to complete 5 years of endocrine therapy
• Tamoxifen for 4.5 to 6 years followed by an aromatase inhibitor for up to 5 years
• Tamoxifen for 4.5 to 6 years then consider to keep taking to complete 10 years of endocrine therapy
• Tamoxifen for 5 years if aromatase inhibitors aren't an option
• Consider tamoxifen for 10 years if aromatase inhibitors aren't an option

6 Endocrine therapy | Regimens

Options for endocrine therapy are based on your menopausal status. All options involve taking an antiestrogen, an aromatase inhibitor, or both back-to-back. These medicines are usually taken for 5 to 10 years. The first regimen received is called the initial treatment. Sometimes a second medicine is taken within the 5-year period. This is called sequential treatment. Endocrine therapy taken beyond the 5-year period is called extended treatment.

Chart 6.2 lists the two options for premenopausal women. The first option is take tamoxifen. Initial treatment with tamoxifen is for 5 years. Ovarian ablation or suppression may be added.

After 5 years of tamoxifen, your menstrual status will be assessed again. If you are still premenopausal, you may stop endocrine therapy or consider taking tamoxifen for another 5 years. If you're postmenopausal, taking an aromatase inhibitor for up to 5 years is advised or consider taking tamoxifen for another 5 years.

The second option for premenopausal women includes ovarian suppression or ablation. This treatment will cause menopause or start a menopause-like phase. An aromatase inhibitor is then taken for 5 years.

Chart 6.3 lists eight options for postmenopausal women. One option is to take an aromatase inhibitor for 5 years. Other options combine the use of an aromatase inhibitor and tamoxifen. In some cases, taking tamoxifen alone is an option. Treatment often lasts for 5 years but sometimes will be taken for 10 years.

Review

- Endocrine therapy is given after surgery to lower the chances of breast cancer returning.

- Endocrine therapy is used to treat only hormone receptor–positive breast cancer.

- For rare cancers that aren't likely to spread outside the breast, endocrine therapy is advised if the breast tumor is larger than 3 cm or the lymph node tumor is larger than 2 mm.

- For breast cancers that have a higher chance of spreading, endocrine therapy is advised unless there is no cancer in lymph nodes.

- There are 4 main types of endocrine therapy. Antiestrogens block the action of estrogen. Aromatase inhibitors, ovarian ablation, and ovarian suppression lower the amount of hormones in the body.

- Which regimens for endocrine therapy are advised is based on menopausal status. Medicines used for endocrine therapy are taken for 5 to 10 years.

- Endocrine therapy causes symptoms of menopause.

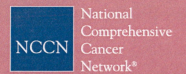

7
Follow-up care

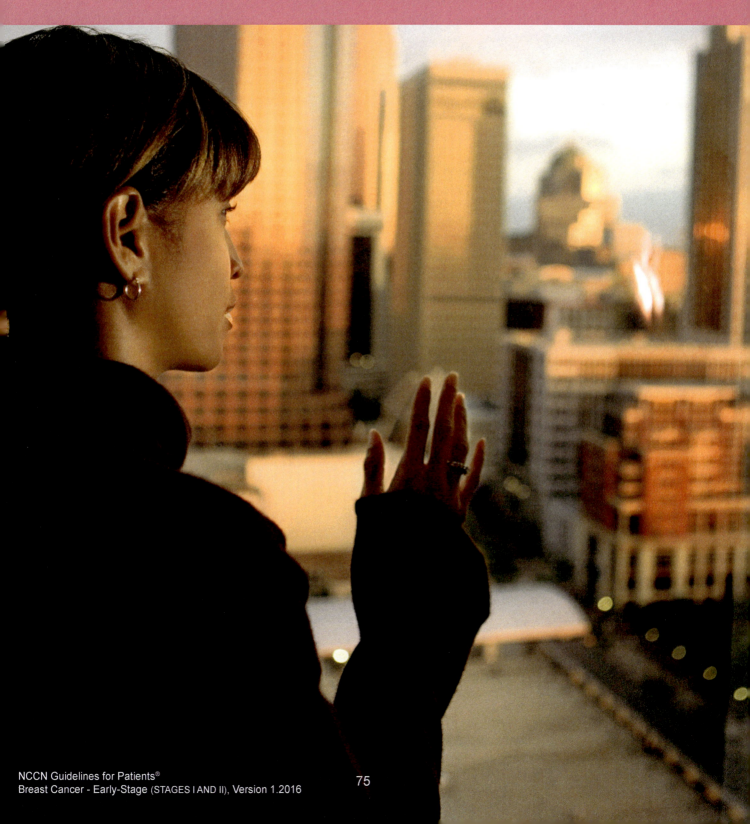

7 Follow-up care

76 Cancer tests
78 Care for side effects
79 Healthy lifestyle
80 Review

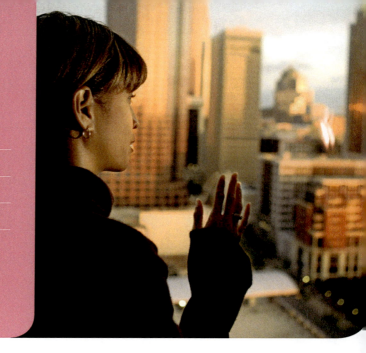

Follow-up care is important. It is done to assess your general health, find new breast tumors early, and check for side effects of treatment. You may still be taking a HER2 inhibitor or endocrine therapy when follow-up care starts.

Cancer tests

Medical history and physical exam
As noted in Chart 7.1, a medical history and physical exam are needed after cancer treatment is finished. Your doctor will take a history and do an exam at follow-up visits. These visits should occur between 1 and 4 times a year as needed for the first 5 years. If results are normal, you should then have these visits every year starting in the 6th year after cancer treatment.

During your visit with your doctor, tell him or her about any new or worse symptoms you have. There may be ways to get relief. If there are changes in your family history of cancer, you should tell your doctor, who may refer you to a genetic counselor.

7 Follow-up care | Cancer tests

Imaging tests

A mammogram should be done each year after lumpectomy or breast-conserving therapy. If you had radiation, your first mammogram should be at least 6 months after you complete radiation. Mammograms can also be used to screen for cancer in a breast that hasn't had cancer. In contrast, mammograms aren't needed if you had your breasts removed by mastectomy. Likewise, imaging of reconstructed breasts on a regular basis isn't needed. Screening for metastases with imaging and lab tests isn't needed unless signs or symptoms that suggest there's cancer appear.

Chart 7.1 Long-term health care

Type of care	Schedule of care
Medical history and physical exam	• Between 1–4 times a year as needed for the first 5 years after treatment ◦ If results are normal, then repeat every year starting in the 6th year after treatment
Mammogram	• If you had radiation therapy, start 6–12 months after radiation ends and repeat test every 12 months • If you didn't have radiation therapy, every 12 months
Lab and imaging tests for metastases	• If signs and symptoms appear
Adherence check	• On a regular basis
GYN exam if: • Taking tamoxifen, and • Uterus is intact	• Every 12 months
Bone mineral density test if: • Taking aromatase inhibitor, or • Treatment-related menopause	• Baseline test then get tested on a regular basis
Lymphedema care	• As needed
Healthy lifestyle	• As often as you can

7 Follow-up care | Care for side effects

Care for side effects

Adherence check
If you take endocrine therapy, it is very important that you don't stop taking your medication. If you do, the cancer will be more likely to return. Tell your doctor about any side effects that make you think about quitting. There may be ways to get relief.

GYN exam
If you take tamoxifen, a GYN (**gyn**ecologic) exam is needed each year since this drug can increase your chances for cancer of the uterus. For this exam, your doctor will ask about any abnormal bleeding. If you have seen any vaginal bleeding that isn't normal for you, tell your doctor.

Bone mineral density
If you take an aromatase inhibitor, you should have your bone mineral density tested regularly. Your bone mineral density should also be tested if cancer treatments caused you to start menopause. Aromatase inhibitors and starting menopause early can cause bone loss. Bone mineral density tests show your doctors how strong your bones are. These tests use x-rays.

Lymphedema
Lymphedema is swelling due to buildup of lymph fluid. It occurs in the arms after lymph node removal. It can happen just after surgery or months to years later if ever. Thus, it's important to know about this side effect so you won't be caught off-guard. If you have lymphedema, your doctor will assess it at follow-up visits and refer you to an expert in lymphedema management. You may be able to reduce the swelling by exercise, massage, and other means.

Healthy lifestyle

Physical activity
Starting or maintaining an active lifestyle is advised. Physical activity has been linked to better treatment results. Ask your treatment team about ways for you to be more active.

Healthy body weight
Like physical activity, a healthy body weight has been linked to better treatment results. BMI (**b**ody **m**ass **i**ndex) is a measure of body fat based on height and weight. A BMI score of 20 to 25 is recommended in order to have the best overall health and breast cancer outcomes. Ask your treatment team about ways to achieve a healthy body weight.

Healthy diet
Healthy eating includes eating a balanced diet, eating the right amount of food, and drinking enough fluids. Healthy eating and limiting your use of alcohol may improve treatment results. You may have special food needs during and after treatment. A nutritionist—an expert in creating a healthy diet—can help.

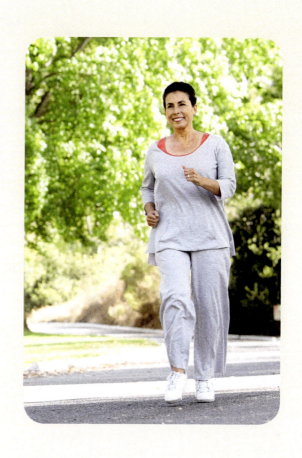

7 Follow-up care | Review

Review

- A medical history, physical exam, and mammograms are advised during follow-up care.

- If you are taking endocrine therapy, it is important that you don't stop until your doctor says you can.

- Getting GYN exams and bone mineral density tests are important if on certain types of endocrine therapy.

- There are ways to reduce swelling from lymphedema.

- Be active, keep a healthy body weight, and eat healthfully.

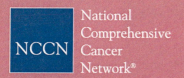

8 Breast cancer recurrence

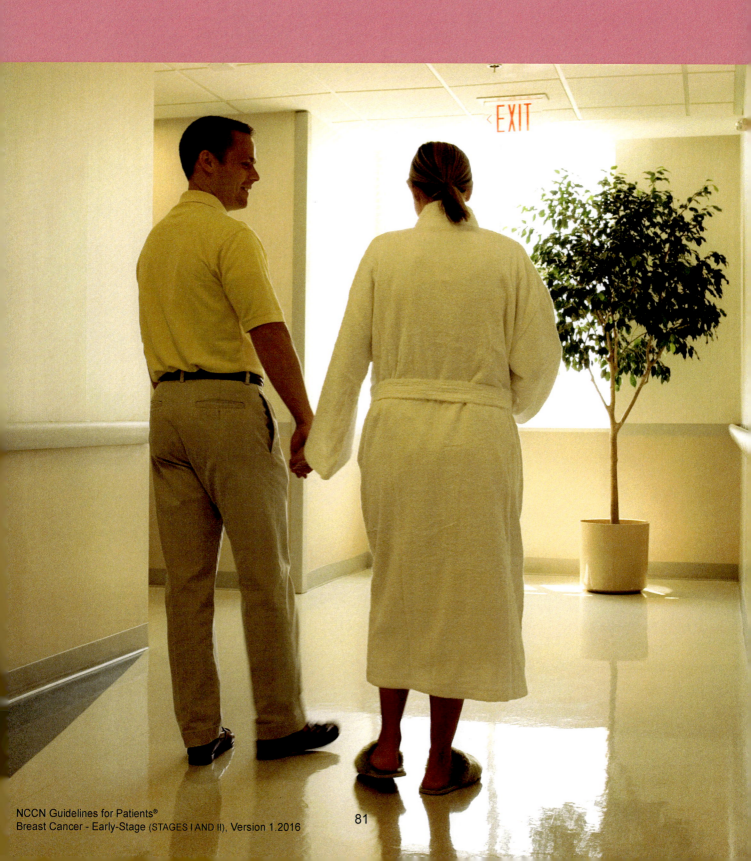

8 Breast cancer recurrence

82 Treatment planning
84 Treatment options
86 Review

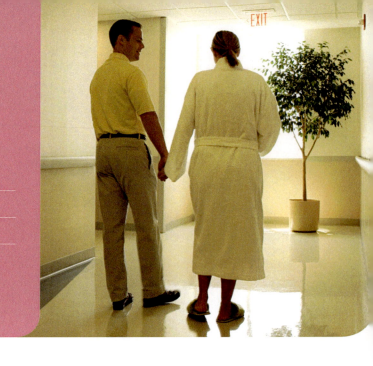

For some women, breast cancer returns after a cancer-free period. Breast cancer may return in or near the breast, near to where a breast was removed, or in distant sites. If the breast cancer returns in distant sites, read the *NCCN Guidelines for Patients®: Breast Cancer - Metastatic Disease (STAGE IV)*. Part 8 discusses treatment for cancer that returns in a breast or near to where a breast is or was.

Treatment planning

Many of the tests that were described in Part 2 are given if the cancer returns. See Chart 8.1. Such tests include a medical history, physical exam, and imaging and blood tests. Genetic counseling is also advised if you have not been tested and hereditary breast cancer is likely.

In addition to the tests in Part 2, other tests may be needed for a recurrence. A biopsy of the recurrence site is advised to confirm there's cancer. The methods for the biopsy depend on the site. The imaging tests described next may also be needed.

Brain MRI
MRI is very useful for viewing the brain. You may have an MRI if you have symptoms that suggest the cancer has spread to the brain. Symptoms of cancer in the brain include chronic headaches, seizures, loss of balance, difficulty walking, speech problems, changes in vision, weakness on one side of the body, and personality changes.

PET/CT

Instead of a bone scan, another way to image bones is by the use of both PET (**p**ositron **e**mission **t**omography) and CT scans. Some cancer centers have an imaging machine that does both scans. At other centers, the scans are done with two machines.

Like a bone scan, PET also uses a radiotracer to see the activity of cells. The radiotracer used to image bone with PET is sodium fluoride. Sodium fluoride PET/CT is a costly test but shows sites of bone damage and repair better than a bone scan. It also has a shorter waiting time of 40 to 60 minutes for the radiotracer to be seen and a shorter scanning time of 15 to 20 minutes than a bone scan.

Another imaging test that is used to see if breast cancer has spread is FDG (**f**luoro**d**eoxy**g**lucose) PET/CT. FDG PET/CT is most helpful when other imaging tests are unclear. It may be helpful with finding breast cancer that has spread to lymph nodes or distant sites.

FDG is a radiotracer that is made of fluoride and a simple form of sugar called glucose. Cancer cells use more FDG than normal cells and thus show up as bright spots on pictures. For this test, you must fast for 4 hours or more.

Bone x-rays

X-rays of bones that hurt are advised. Long and weight-bearing bones that aren't normal on bone scan or PET/CT should also be x-rayed. During an x-ray, you must lie still on a table while the x-ray machine sends small amounts of radiation into your body. Images made from the x-rays are seen on a screen.

Chart 8.1 Health care before recurrence treatment

Main tests and services	Other care based on signs and symptoms
• Medical history	• MRI scan if CNS symptoms start
• Physical exam	• X-rays of bones that hurt
• Chest diagnostic CT	• X-rays of long or weight-bearing bones that are abnormal on bone scan
• Abdominal ± pelvic diagnostic CT or MRI	
• Bone scan or sodium fluoride PET/CT	
• FDG PET/CT is an option	
• Complete blood count	
• Liver function tests	
• Biopsy of recurrence site	
• Hormone and HER2 receptor tests on metastatic sites	
• Genetic counseling if hereditary breast cancer is likely	

Treatment options

Chart 8.2 Local recurrence only

Prior treatment	What treatment should I have?
• Breast-conserving therapy	• Total mastectomy, • Axillary lymph node dissection, and • Consider systemic treatment
• Total mastectomy	• Surgery if possible, • Radiation therapy to the chest wall and supraclavicular and infraclavicular areas, and • Consider systemic treatment
• Total mastectomy, • Axillary lymph node dissection, and • Radiation therapy	• Surgery if possible, and • Consider systemic treatment

Chart 8.3 Lymph node recurrence

Lymph node site	What treatment should I have?
• Axillary lymph nodes	• Surgery, • Radiation therapy to the chest wall, axilla, and supraclavicular and infraclavicular nodes, and • Consider systemic treatment
• Supraclavicular lymph nodes	• Radiation therapy to the chest wall and supraclavicular and infraclavicular nodes, and • Consider systemic treatment
• Internal mammary lymph nodes	• Radiation therapy to the chest wall, supraclavicular and infraclavicular areas, and internal mammary nodes, and • Consider systemic treatment

8 Breast cancer recurrence | Treatment options

Treatment options are based in part on where the recurrence is. A local recurrence is breast cancer that returned within a breast or within the chest wall near to where a breast is or was. A regional recurrence includes breast cancer that returned in lymph nodes near to the breast area. These lymph nodes include those near your armpit (axillary lymph nodes), below your collarbone (infraclavicular lymph nodes), above your collarbone (supraclavicular lymph nodes), and near to your breastbone (internal mammary nodes).

Treatment options for recurrences are explained next. Doctors use the term "systemic" when talking about a cancer treatment for the whole body. Systemic treatment for breast cancer recurrences includes chemotherapy, chemotherapy with HER2 inhibitors, and endocrine therapy.

Chart 8.2 lists the treatment options for a local recurrence based on your prior treatment. If you had breast-conserving therapy, a total mastectomy is advised. You may also have an axillary lymph node dissection if not done before. Systemic treatment may be part of your treatment, too.

If previously treated with mastectomy alone, you may have surgery to remove the cancer. Afterward, radiation therapy to the chest wall and the lymph nodes around your collarbone is advised. Systemic treatment may be added.

You may have had a mastectomy, axillary lymph node dissection, and radiation therapy. In this case, the cancer should be removed by surgery if possible. Systemic treatment may be added.

Chart 8.3 lists the treatment options for a recurrence in your lymph nodes. The cancer may have also returned in or near a breast. Treatment options are based on which lymph nodes have cancer.

If cancer is found in your axillary lymph nodes, these lymph nodes should be removed if possible. Radiation therapy is also advised. Radiation sites include your chest wall, near your armpit (axilla), and the lymph nodes around your collarbone. You may receive systemic treatment, too.

Radiation therapy without surgery is advised for the return of cancer in supraclavicular or internal mammary nodes. For a supraclavicular recurrence, radiation sites include your chest wall and lymph nodes around the collarbone. For an internal mammary recurrence, radiation sites include your chest wall, internal mammary nodes, and nodes around the collarbone. You may receive systemic treatment, too.

8 Breast cancer recurrence | Review

Review

- Breast cancer may return in or near the breast, near to where the breast was removed, or in distant organs.

- Treatment planning is needed for a recurrence.

- Treatment for a local recurrence is based on prior treatment. Surgery is advised if possible. Treatment should also include radiation therapy if not received before. Systemic treatment may be part of your treatment.

- Treatment for a recurrence in your lymph nodes depends on which lymph nodes have cancer. Surgery with radiation therapy is advised for a recurrence in axillary lymph nodes. Recurrences in other lymph nodes should be treated with radiation therapy. Systemic treatment may be received after any type of lymph node recurrence.

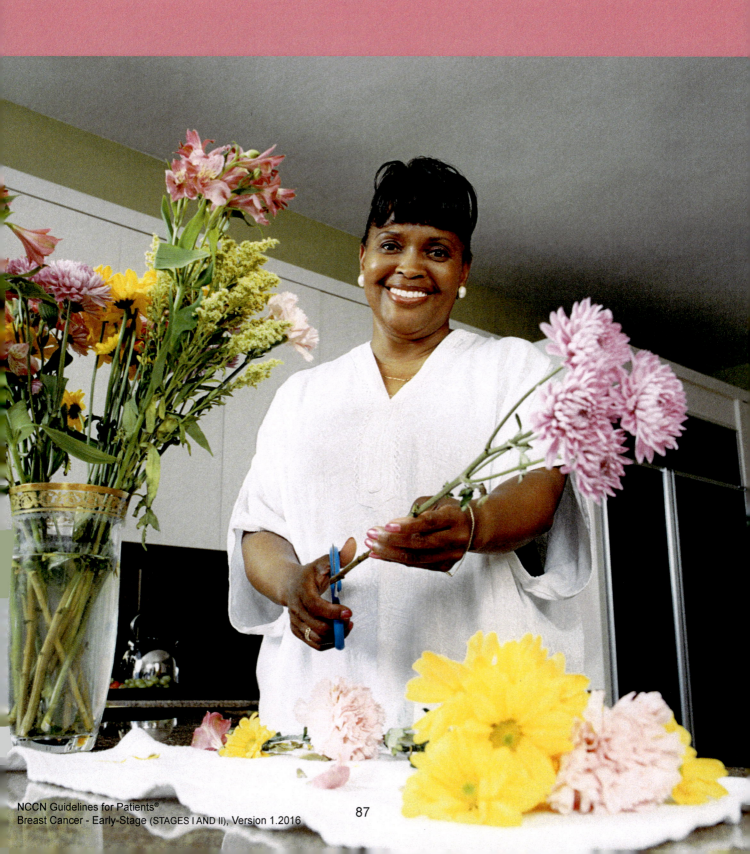

9 Making treatment decisions

9 Making treatment decisions

- 89 It's your choice
- 90 Questions to ask your doctors
- 94 Weighing your options
- 96 Websites
- 96 Review

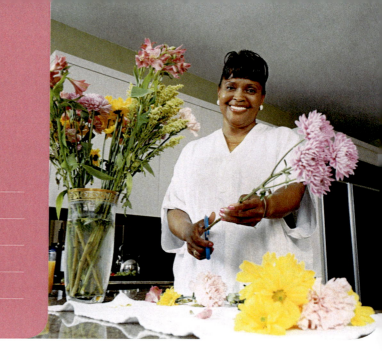

Having cancer is very stressful. While absorbing the fact that you have cancer, you have to learn about tests and treatments. In addition, the time you have to accept a treatment plan feels short. Parts 1 through 8 described the cancer and the test and treatment options recommended by NCCN experts. These options are based on science and agreement among NCCN experts. Part 9 aims to help you make decisions that are in line with your beliefs, wishes, and values.

It's your choice

The role patients want in choosing their treatment differs. You may feel uneasy about making treatment decisions. This may be due to a high level of stress. It may be hard to hear or know what others are saying. Stress, pain, and drugs can limit your ability to make good decisions. You may feel uneasy because you don't know much about cancer. You've never heard the words used to describe cancer, tests, or treatments. Likewise, you may think that your judgment isn't any better than your doctors'.

Letting others decide which option is best may make you feel more at ease. But, whom do you want to make the decisions? You may rely on your doctors alone to make the right decisions. However, your doctors may not tell you which to choose if you have multiple good options. You can also have loved ones help. They can gather information, speak on your behalf, and share in decision-making with your doctors. Even if others decide which treatment you will receive, you still have to agree by signing a consent form.

On the other hand, you may want to take the lead or share in decision-making. Most patients do. In shared decision-making, you and your doctors share information, weigh the options, and agree on a treatment plan. Your doctors know the science behind your plan but you know your concerns and goals. By working together, you are likely to get a higher quality of care and be more satisfied. You'll likely get the treatment you want, at the place you want, and by the doctors you want.

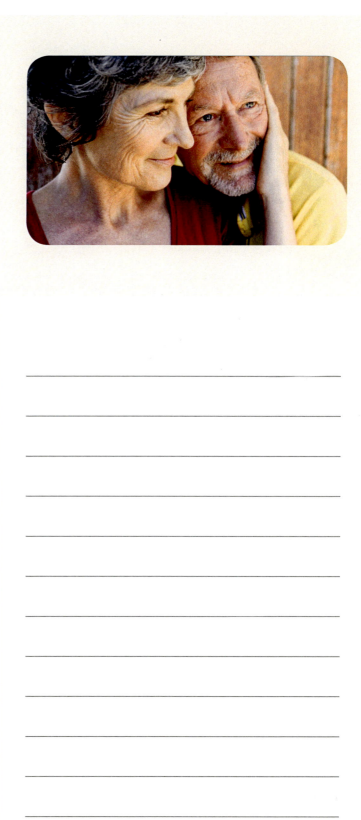

9 Making treatment decisions | Questions to ask your doctors

Questions to ask your doctors

You may meet with experts from different fields of medicine. Strive to have helpful talks with each person. Prepare questions before your visit and ask questions if the person isn't clear. You can also record your talks and get copies of your medical records. It may be helpful to have your spouse, partner, family member, or a friend with you at these visits. A patient advocate or navigator might also be able to come. They can help to ask questions and remember what was said. Suggested questions to ask include:

What's my diagnosis and prognosis?

It's important to know that there are different types of cancer. Cancer can greatly differ even when people have a tumor in the same organ. Based on your test results, your doctors can tell you which type of cancer you have. He or she can also give a prognosis. A prognosis is a prediction of the pattern and outcome of a disease. Knowing the prognosis may affect what you decide about treatment.

1. Where did the cancer start? In what type of cell?
2. Is this cancer common?
3. What is the cancer stage? Does this stage mean the cancer has spread far?
4. Is this a fast- or slow-growing breast cancer?
5. What other tests results are important to know?
6. How often are these tests wrong?
7. Would you give me a copy of the pathology report and other test results?
8. How likely is it that I'll be cancer-free after treatment?

9 Making treatment decisions | Questions to ask your doctors

What are my options?

There is no single treatment practice that is best for all patients. There is often more than one treatment option along with clinical trial options. Your doctor will review your test results and recommend treatment options.

1. What will happen if I do nothing?
2. Can I just carefully monitor the cancer?
3. Do you consult NCCN recommendations when considering options?
4. Are you suggesting options other than what NCCN recommends? If yes, why?
5. Do your suggested options include clinical trials? Please explain why.
6. How do my age, health, and other factors affect my options?
7. What if I am pregnant?
8. Which option is proven to work best?
9. Which options lack scientific proof?
10. What are the benefits of each option? Does any option offer a cure? Are my chances any better for one option than another? Less time-consuming? Less expensive?
11. What are the risks of each option? What are possible complications? What are the rare and common side effects? Short-lived and long-lasting side effects? Serious or mild side effects? Other risks?
12. What can be done to prevent or relieve the side effects of treatment?
13. What are my chances that the cancer will return?
14. What are my options for breast reconstruction?

_____

_____

_____

_____

9 Making treatment decisions | Questions to ask your doctors

What does each option require of me?

Many patients consider how each option will practically affect their lives. This information may be important because you have family, jobs, and other duties to take care of. You also may be concerned about getting the help you need. If you have more than one option, choosing the option that is the least taxing may be important to you:

1. Will I have to go to the hospital or elsewhere? How often? How long is each visit?
2. Do I have a choice of when to begin treatment? Can I choose the days and times of treatment?
3. How do I prepare for treatment? Do I have to stop taking any of my medicines? Are there foods I will have to avoid?
4. Should I bring someone with me when I get treated?
5. Will the treatment hurt?
6. How much will the treatment cost me? What does my insurance cover?
7. Will I miss work or school? Will I be able to drive?
8. Is home care after treatment needed? If yes, what type?
9. How soon will I be able to manage my own health?
10. When will I be able to return to my normal activities?

9 Making treatment decisions | Questions to ask your doctors

What is your experience?

More and more research is finding that patients treated by more experienced doctors have better results. It is important to learn if a doctor is an expert in the cancer treatment he or she is offering.

1. Are you board certified? If yes, in what area?
2. How many patients like me have you treated?
3. How many procedures like the one you're suggesting have you done?
4. Is this treatment a major part of your practice?
5. How many of your patients have had complications?

9 Making treatment decisions | Weighing your options

Weighing your options

Deciding which option is best can be hard. Doctors from different fields of medicine may have different opinions on which option is best for you. This can be very confusing. Your spouse or partner may disagree with which option you want. This can be stressful. In some cases, one option hasn't been shown to work better than another, so science isn't helpful. Some ways to decide on treatment are discussed next.

2nd opinion

The time around a cancer diagnosis is very stressful. People with cancer often want to get treated as soon as possible. They want to make their cancer go away before it spreads farther. While cancer can't be ignored, there is time to think about and choose which option is best for you.

You may wish to have another doctor review your test results and suggest a treatment plan. This is called getting a 2nd opinion. You may completely trust your doctor, but a 2nd opinion on which option is best can help.

Copies of the pathology report, a DVD of the imaging tests, and other test results need to be sent to the doctor giving the 2nd opinion. Some people feel uneasy asking for copies from their doctors. However, a 2nd opinion is a normal part of cancer care.

When doctors have cancer, most will talk with more than one doctor before choosing their treatment. What's more, some health plans require a 2nd opinion. If your health plan doesn't cover the cost of a 2nd opinion, you have the choice of paying for it yourself.

If the two opinions are the same, you may feel more at peace about the treatment you accept to have. If the two opinions differ, think about getting a 3rd opinion. A 3rd opinion may help you decide between your options. Choosing your cancer treatment is a very important decision. It can affect your length and quality of life.

Decision aids

Decision aids are tools that help people make complex choices. For example, you may have to choose between two options that work equally as well. Sometimes making a decision is hard because there is a lack of science supporting a treatment.

Decision aids often focus on one decision point. In contrast, this book presents tests and treatment options at each point of care for women in general. Well-designed decision aids include information that research has identified as what people need to make decisions. They also aim to help you think about what's important based on your values and preferences.

A listing of decision aids can be found at decisionaid.ohri.ca/AZlist.html. Decision aids specific to stages I and II breast cancer are:

Genetic testing:
www.uofmhealth.org/health-library/zx3000

Breast-conserving therapy vs. mastectomy:
www.uofmhealth.org/health-library/tv6530#zx3718

Breast reconstruction after mastectomy:
www.uofmhealth.org/health-library/tb1934#zx3672

Support groups

Besides talking to health experts, it may help to talk to patients who have walked in your shoes. Support groups often consist of people at different stages of treatment. Some may be in the process of deciding while others may be finished with treatment. At support groups, you can ask questions and hear about the experiences of other women with breast cancer.

9 Making treatment decisions | Weighing your options

Compare benefits and downsides

Every option has benefits and downsides. Consider these when deciding which option is best for you. Talking to others can help identify benefits and downsides you haven't thought of. Scoring each factor from 0 to 10 can also help since some factors may be more important to you than others.

Websites

American Cancer Society
www.cancer.org/cancer/breastcancer/index

National Coalition for Cancer Survivorship
www.canceradvocacy.org/toolbox

National Cancer Institute
www.cancer.gov/types/breast

NCCN
www.nccn.org/patients

Breast Cancer Alliance
www.breastcanceralliance.org

FORCE: Facing Our Risk of Cancer Empowered
www.facingourrisk.org

Living Beyond Breast Cancer
www.lbbc.org

Sharsharet
www.sharsheret.org

Young Survival Coalition (YSC)
youngsurvival.org

Rockin' for the Cure®
www.rockinforthecure.net

Review

- Shared decision-making is a process in which you and your doctors plan treatment together.

- Asking your doctors questions is vital to getting the information you need to make informed decisions.

- Getting a 2nd opinion, using decision aids, attending support groups, and comparing benefits and downsides may help you decide which treatment is best for you.

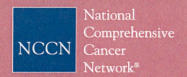

Glossary

Dictionary

Acronyms

Dictionary

abdomen
The belly area between the chest and pelvis.

adjuvant treatment
Treatment that is given to lower the chances of the cancer returning.

adrenal gland
A small organ on top of each kidney that makes hormones.

alkaline phosphatase (ALP)
A protein found in most tissues of the body.

antiestrogen
A drug that stops estrogen from attaching to cells.

aromatase inhibitor
A drug that lowers the level of estrogen in the body.

axillary lymph node
A small group of special disease-fighting cells located near the armpit.

axillary lymph node dissection
Surgery to remove axillary lymph nodes.

bilateral diagnostic mammogram
A test that uses multiple x-rays to make pictures of the insides of both breasts.

biopsy
Removal of small amounts of tissue or fluid to be tested for disease.

bone mineral density
A test that measures the strength of bones.

bone scan
A test that uses radioactive material to assess for bone damage.

boost
An extra dose of radiation to a specific area of the body.

breast implant
A small bag filled with salt water, gel, or both that is used to remake breasts.

breast reconstruction
Surgery to rebuild breasts.

breast-conserving therapy
Cancer treatment that includes removing the breast lump and radiation therapy.

cancer stage
Rating of the growth and spread of tumors.

carcinoma
Cancer that starts in cells that form the lining of organs and structures in the body.

catheter
A flexible tube inserted in the body to give treatment or drain fluid from the body.

chemotherapy
Drugs that stop the life cycle of cells so they don't increase in number.

chest wall
The layer of muscle, bone, and tissue on the outer part of the chest.

clinical breast exam
A physical exam of the breasts by a health professional to feel for disease.

clinical stage
The rating of the extent of cancer based on tests before treatment.

clinical trial
Research on a test or treatment to assess its safety or how well it works.

complete blood count (CBC)
A test of the number of blood cells.

computed tomography (CT)
A test that uses x-rays from many angles to make a picture of the inside of the body.

contrast
A dye put into your body to make clearer pictures during imaging tests.

core needle biopsy
Use of a needle to remove a large tissue sample to test for cancer cells.

Glossary

deoxyribonucleic acid (DNA)
A very thin and long molecule that contains genetic code. Also called the "blueprint of life."

duct
A tube in the breast that drains breast milk.

ductal carcinoma
A breast cancer that starts in a cell that lines the ducts of the breast.

endocrine therapy
Treatment that stops the making or action of hormones in the body. Also called hormone therapy.

estrogen
A hormone that develops female body traits.

external beam radiation therapy (EBRT)
Treatment with radiation received from a machine outside the body.

fertility specialist
An expert who helps women to have babies.

fine-needle aspiration (FNA)
Removal of a small tissue sample with a very thin needle.

flap
Tissue taken from one area of the body and used in another area.

follicle-stimulating hormone (FSH)
A hormone made by the ovaries.

gene
Coded instructions in cells for making new cells and controlling how cells behave.

general anesthesia
A controlled loss of wakefulness from drugs.

genetic counseling
Discussion with a health expert about the risk for a disease caused by changes in genes.

hereditary breast cancer
Breast cancer caused by faulty, coded information in cells that was passed down from parent to child.

hormone
Chemical in the body that activates cells or organs.

Dictionary

hormone receptor–negative
Cancer cells that don't use hormones to grow.

hormone receptor–positive
Cancer cells that use hormones to grow.

human epidermal growth factor receptor 2 (HER2)
A protein on the edge of a cell that send signals for the cell to grow.

human epidermal growth factor receptor 2 (HER2) inhibitor
A cancer drug that stops the effect of a cell protein called HER2.

human epidermal growth factor receptor 2 (HER2)-negative
Cancer cells with normal numbers of HER2 receptors.

human epidermal growth factor receptor 2 (HER2)-positive
Cancer cells with too many HER2 receptors.

imaging test
A test that makes pictures of the insides of the body.

immunohistochemistry (IHC)
A lab test of cancer cells to find specific cell traits involved in abnormal cell growth.

in situ hybridization (ISH)
A lab test of that counts the number of copies of a gene.

infraclavicular
The area right below the collarbone.

intensity-modulated radiation therapy (IMRT)
Radiation therapy that uses small beams of different strengths based on the thickness of the tissue.

internal mammary
The area along the breastbone.

internal radiation
Treatment with radiation received from an object placed near or in the tumor. Also called brachytherapy.

invasive breast cancer
Cancer cells have grown into the supporting tissue of the breast.

liver function test
A test that measures chemicals made or processed by the liver.

Glossary / Dictionary

lobular carcinoma
A breast cancer that started in cells that line the breast lobules.

lobule
A gland in the breast that makes breast milk.

local anesthesia
A controlled loss of feeling in a small area of the body from drugs.

lumpectomy
Surgery to remove a breast lump and some normal tissue around it.

luteinizing hormone-releasing hormone (LHRH)
A hormone in the brain that helps control the making of estrogen by the ovaries.

lymph
A clear fluid containing white blood cells.

lymph node
Small groups of special disease-fighting cells located throughout the body.

lymphedema
Swelling of the body due to a buildup of lymph.

magnetic resonance imaging (MRI)
A test that uses a magnetic field and radio waves to make pictures of the insides of the body.

mammogram
A picture of the insides of the breast that is made by an x-ray test.

mastectomy
Surgery to remove the whole breast.

medical history
All health events and medications taken to date.

menopause
The point in time when menstrual periods end.

metaplastic carcinoma
Cancer that changed from one cell type to another.

mixed carcinoma
Cancer that has more than one cell type.

mucinous breast cancer
Cancer that has a lot of mucus around the cells. Also called colloid breast cancer.

multiple-catheter boost radiation
Use of multiple small tubes to place radioactive seeds in your body for treatment.

mutation
An abnormal change in the instructions within cells for making and controlling cells.

neoadjuvant treatment
Treatment given before the main treatment used to cure disease. Also called preoperative treatment.

nipple replacement
The rebuilding of a breast nipple.

noninvasive breast cancer
Cancer cells have not grown into the supporting tissue of the breast.

ovarian ablation
Methods used to stop the ovaries from making hormones.

ovarian suppression
Methods used to lower the amount of hormones made by the ovaries.

partial breast irradiation
Treatment with radiation that is only directed at the surgery site.

pathologic stage
A rating of the extent of cancer based on tests given after treatment.

pathologist
A doctor who's an expert in testing cells and tissue to find disease.

pelvis
The area between the hip bones.

physical exam
A review of the body by a health expert for signs of disease.

positron emission tomography (PET)
Use of radioactive material to see the shape and function of body parts.

postmenopause
The state of the end of menstrual periods.

premenopause
The state of having regular menstrual periods.

progesterone
A hormone in women that is involved in sexual development, periods, and pregnancy.

puberty
The time when teens sexually develop.

radiation therapy
The use of high-energy rays to destroy cancer cells.

receptor
A protein within cells to which substances can attach.

recurrence
The return of cancer after a cancer-free period.

sentinel lymph node
The first lymph node to which cancer cells spread after leaving the breast tumor.

sentinel lymph node biopsy
Surgery to remove the first lymph node(s) to which cancer cells spread after leaving the breast tumor. Also called sentinel lymph node dissection.

side effect
An unplanned physical or emotional response to treatment.

skin-sparing mastectomy
A surgery that removes all breast tissue but saves as much breast skin as possible.

stroma
Supportive tissue in the breast.

supportive care
Treatment for the symptoms or health conditions cause by cancer or cancer treatment.

supraclavicular
The area right above the collarbone.

surgical margin
The normal tissue around the edge of a tumor that is removed during surgery.

total mastectomy
Surgery that removes the entire breast but no chest muscles. Also called simple mastectomy.

tubular breast cancer
Cancer that has cells that look like tubes.

ultrasound
Use of sound waves to make pictures of the insides of the body.

volume displacement
The shifting of breast tissue.

whole breast radiation
Treatment of the entire breast with radiation from a machine outside the body.

Acronyms

AJCC
American Joint Committee on Cancer

ALP
alkaline phosphatase

BMI
body mass index

CBC
complete blood count

cm
centimeters

CT
computed tomography

DNA
deoxyribonucleic acid

EBRT
external beam radiation therapy

FDG
fluorodeoxyglucose

FNA
fine-needle aspiration

FSH
follicle-stimulating hormone

GYN
gynecologic

HER2
human epidermal growth factor receptor 2

IHC
immunohistochemistry

IMRT
intensity-modulated radiation therapy

ISH
in situ hybridization

LHRH
luteinizing hormone-releasing hormone

MRI
magnetic resonance imaging

PET
positron emission tomography

PET/CT
positron emission tomography/ computed tomography

SERM
selective estrogen receptor modulator

VUS
variants of unknown significance

NCCN Abbreviations and Acronyms

NCCN®
National Comprehensive Cancer Network®

NCCN Patient Guidelines
NCCN Guidelines for Patients®

NCCN Guidelines®
NCCN Clinical Practice Guidelines in Oncology®

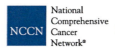

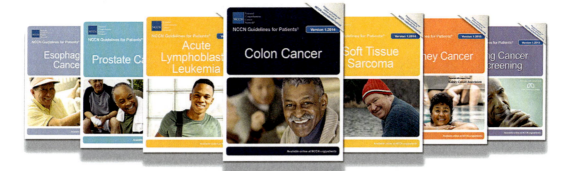

NCCN GUIDELINES FOR PATIENTS®

Patient-friendly versions of the NCCN Clinical Practice Guidelines in Oncology (NCCN Guidelines®)

View and download your free copy ➡ **NCCN.org/patients**

Order print copies ➡ **Amazon.com** *(Search 'NCCN Guidelines for Patients')*

- Acute Lymphoblastic Leukemia
- Caring for Adolescents and Young Adults (AYA)*
- Chronic Lymphocytic Leukemia
- Chronic Myelogenous Leukemia
- Colon Cancer
- Esophageal Cancer
- Hodgkin Lymphoma
- Kidney Cancer
- Lung Cancer Screening
- Malignant Pleural Mesothelioma
- Melanoma
- Multiple Myeloma
- Myelodysplastic Syndromes
- Non-Hodgkin's Lymphomas
  - Diffuse Large B-cell Lymphoma
  - Follicular Lymphoma
  - Mantle Cell Lymphoma
  - Mycosis Fungoides
  - Peripheral T-cell Lymphoma
- Non-Small Cell Lung Cancer
- Ovarian Cancer
- Pancreatic Cancer
- Prostate Cancer
- Soft Tissue Sarcoma
- Stage 0 Breast Cancer
- Stages I and II Breast Cancer
- Stage III Breast Cancer
- Stage IV Breast Cancer

The NCCN Guidelines for Patients® are supported by charitable donations made to the NCCN Foundation®

DONATE NOW
nccnfoundation.org

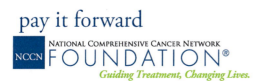

NEW!
NCCN Quick Guide™ Sheets

Key points from the complete NCCN Guidelines for Patients

Visit NCCN.org/patients for free access

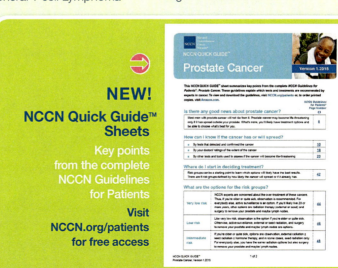

* Print copies unavailable at this time. Check NCCN.org/patients for updates.

As of May 12, 2016

NCCN.org – For Clinicians | **NCCN.org/patients** – For Patients

State Fundraising Notices

FLORIDA: A COPY OF THE OFFICIAL REGISTRATION AND FINANCIAL INFORMATION OF NCCN FOUNDATION MAY BE OBTAINED FROM THE DIVISION OF CONSUMER SERVICES BY CALLING TOLL-FREE WITHIN THE STATE 1-800-HELP-FLA. REGISTRATION DOES NOT IMPLY ENDORSEMENT, APPROVAL, OR RECOMMENDATION BY THE STATE. FLORIDA REGISTRATION #CH33263. **GEORGIA:** The following information will be sent upon request: (A) A full and fair description of the programs and activities of NCCN Foundation; and (B) A financial statement or summary which shall be consistent with the financial statement required to be filed with the Secretary of State pursuant to Code Section 43-17-5. **KANSAS:** The annual financial report for NCCN Foundation, 275 Commerce Drive, Suite 300, Fort Washington, PA 19034, 215-690-0300, State Registration # 445-497-1, is filed with the Secretary of State. **MARYLAND:** A copy of the NCCN Foundation financial report is available by calling NCCN Foundation at 215-690-0300 or writing to 275 Commerce Drive, Suite 300, Fort Washington, PA 19034. For the cost of copying and postage, documents and information filed under the Maryland charitable organizations law can be obtained from the Secretary of State, Charitable Division, State House, Annapolis, MD 21401, 1-410-974-5534. **MICHIGAN:** Registration Number MICS 45298. **MISSISSIPPI:** The official registration and financial information of NCCN Foundation may be obtained from the Mississippi Secretary of State's office by calling 888-236-6167. Registration by the Secretary of State does not imply endorsement by the Secretary of State. **NEW JERSEY:** INFORMATION FILED WITH THE ATTORNEY GENERAL CONCERNING THIS CHARITABLE SOLICITATION AND THE PERCENTAGE OF CONTRIBUTIONS RECEIVED BY THE CHARITY DURING THE LAST REPORTING PERIOD THAT WERE DEDICATED TO THE CHARITABLE PURPOSE MAY BE OBTAINED FROM THE ATTORNEY GENERAL OF THE STATE OF NEW JERSEY BY CALLING (973) 504-6215 AND IS AVAILABLE ON THE INTERNET AT www.njconsumeraffairs.gov/ocp.htm#charity. REGISTRATION WITH THE ATTORNEY GENERAL DOES NOT IMPLY ENDORSEMENT. **NEW YORK:** A copy of the latest annual report may be obtained from NCCN Foundation, 275 Commerce Drive, Suite 300, Fort Washington, PA 19034, or the Charities Bureau, Department of Law. 120 Broadway, New York, NY 10271. **NORTH CAROLINA: FINANCIAL INFORMATION ABOUT THIS ORGANIZATION AND A COPY OF ITS LICENSE ARE AVAILABLE FROM THE STATE SOLICITATION LICENSING BRANCH AT 888-830-4989 (within North Carolina) or (919) 807-2214 (outside of North Carolina). THE LICENSE IS NOT AN ENDORSEMENT BY THE STATE. PENNSYLVANIA:** The official registration and financial information of NCCN Foundation may be obtained from the Pennsylvania Department of State by calling toll-free within Pennsylvania, 800-732-0999. Registration does not imply endorsement. **VIRGINIA:** A financial statement for the most recent fiscal year is available upon request from the State Division of Consumer Affairs, P.O. Box 1163, Richmond, VA 23218; 1-804-786-1343. **WASHINGTON:** Our charity is registered with the Secretary of State and information relating to our financial affairs is available from the Secretary of State, toll free for Washington residents 800-332-4483. **WEST VIRGINIA:** West Virginia residents may obtain a summary of the registration and financial documents from the Secretary of State, State Capitol, Charleston, WV 25305. Registration does not imply endorsement.

Consult with the IRS or your tax professional regarding tax deductibility. REGISTRATION OR LICENSING WITH A STATE AGENCY DOES NOT CONSTITUTE OR IMPLY ENDORSEMENT, APPROVAL, OR RECOMMENDATION BY THAT STATE. We care about your privacy and how we communicate with you, and how we use and share your information. For a copy of NCCN Foundation's Privacy Policy, please call 215.690.0300 or visit our website at **www.nccn.org**.

NCCN Panel Members for Breast Cancer

William J. Gradishar, MD/Chair
Robert H. Lurie Comprehensive Cancer Center of Northwestern University

Benjamin O. Anderson, MD/Vice-Chair
Fred Hutchinson Cancer Research Center/Seattle Cancer Care Alliance

Ron Balassanian, MD
UCSF Helen Diller Family Comprehensive Cancer Center

Sarah L. Blair, MD
UC San Diego Moores Cancer Center

Harold J. Burstein, MD, PhD
Dana-Farber/Brigham and Women's Cancer Center

Amy Cyr, MD
Siteman Cancer Center at Barnes-Jewish Hospital and Washington University School of Medicine

Anthony D. Elias, MD
University of Colorado Cancer Center

William B. Farrar, MD
The Ohio State University Comprehensive Cancer Center - James Cancer Hospital and Solove Research Institute

Andres Forero, MD
University of Alabama at Birmingham Comprehensive Cancer Center

Sharon Hermes Giordano, MD, MPH
The University of Texas MD Anderson Cancer Center

Matthew Goetz, MD
Mayo Clinic Cancer Center

Lori J. Goldstein, MD
Fox Chase Cancer Center

Clifford A. Hudis, MD
Memorial Sloan Kettering Cancer Center

Steven J. Isakoff, MD, PhD
Massachusetts General Hospital Cancer Center

P. Kelly Marcom, MD
Duke Cancer Institute

Ingrid A. Mayer, MD
Vanderbilt-Ingram Cancer Center

Beryl McCormick, MD
Memorial Sloan Kettering Cancer Center

Meena Moran, MD
Yale Cancer Center/Smilow Cancer Hospital

Sameer A. Patel, MD
Fox Chase Cancer Center

Lori J. Pierce, MD
University of Michigan Comprehensive Cancer Center

Elizabeth C. Reed, MD
Fred & Pamela Buffett Cancer Center

Kilian E. Salerno, MD
Roswell Park Cancer Institute

Lee S. Schwartzberg, MD
St. Jude Children's Research Hospital/ The University of Tennessee Health Science Center

Karen Lisa Smith, MD, MPH
The Sidney Kimmel Comprehensive Cancer Center at Johns Hopkins

Mary Lou Smith, JD, MBA
Research Advocacy Network Patient Advocate

Hatem Soliman, MD
Moffitt Cancer Center

George Somlo, MD
City of Hope Comprehensive Cancer Center

Melinda Telli, MD
Stanford Cancer Institute

John H. Ward, MD
Huntsman Cancer Institute at the University of Utah

NCCN Staff

Dorothy A. Shead, MS
Director, Patient and Clinical Information Operations

Rashmi Kumar, PhD
Senior Medical Writer

For disclosures, visit www.nccn.org/about/disclosure.aspx.

NCCN Member Institutions

Fred & Pamela Buffett Cancer Center
Omaha, Nebraska
800.999.5465
nebraskamed.com/cancer

Case Comprehensive Cancer Center/
University Hospitals Seidman
Cancer Center and Cleveland Clinic
Taussig Cancer Institute
Cleveland, Ohio
800.641.2422 • UH Seidman Cancer Center
uhhospitals.org/seidman
866.223.8100 • CC Taussig Cancer Institute
my.clevelandclinic.org/services/cancer
216.844.8797 • Case CCC
case.edu/cancer

City of Hope Comprehensive
Cancer Center
Los Angeles, California
800.826.4673
cityofhope.org

Dana-Farber/Brigham and
Women's Cancer Center
Massachusetts General Hospital
Cancer Center
Boston, Massachusetts
877.332.4294
dfbwcc.org
massgeneral.org/cancer

Duke Cancer Institute
Durham, North Carolina
888.275.3853
dukecancerinstitute.org

Fox Chase Cancer Center
Philadelphia, Pennsylvania
888.369.2427
foxchase.org

Huntsman Cancer Institute
at the University of Utah
Salt Lake City, Utah
877.585.0303
huntsmancancer.org

Fred Hutchinson Cancer
Research Center/
Seattle Cancer Care Alliance
Seattle, Washington
206.288.7222 • seattlecca.org
206.667.5000 • fredhutch.org

The Sidney Kimmel Comprehensive
Cancer Center at Johns Hopkins
Baltimore, Maryland
410.955.8964
hopkinskimmelcancercenter.org

Robert H. Lurie Comprehensive Cancer
Center of Northwestern University
Chicago, Illinois
866.587.4322
cancer.northwestern.edu

Mayo Clinic Cancer Center
Phoenix/Scottsdale, Arizona
Jacksonville, Florida
Rochester, Minnesota
800.446.2279 • Arizona
904.953.0853 • Florida
507.538.3270 • Minnesota
mayoclinic.org/departments-centers/mayo-clinic-cancer-center

Memorial Sloan Kettering
Cancer Center
New York, New York
800.525.2225
mskcc.org

Moffitt Cancer Center
Tampa, Florida
800.456.3434
moffitt.org

The Ohio State University
Comprehensive Cancer Center -
James Cancer Hospital and
Solove Research Institute
Columbus, Ohio
800.293.5066
cancer.osu.edu

Roswell Park Cancer Institute
Buffalo, New York
877.275.7724
roswellpark.org

Siteman Cancer Center at Barnes-
Jewish Hospital and Washington
University School of Medicine
St. Louis, Missouri
800.600.3606
siteman.wustl.edu

St. Jude Children's Research Hospital/
The University of Tennessee
Health Science Center
Memphis, Tennessee
888.226.4343 • stjude.org
901.683.0055 • westclinic.com

Stanford Cancer Institute
Stanford, California
877.668.7535
cancer.stanford.edu

University of Alabama at Birmingham
Comprehensive Cancer Center
Birmingham, Alabama
800.822.0933
www3.ccc.uab.edu

UC San Diego Moores Cancer Center
La Jolla, California
858.657.7000
cancer.ucsd.edu

UCSF Helen Diller Family
Comprehensive Cancer Center
San Francisco, California
800.689.8273
cancer.ucsf.edu

University of Colorado Cancer Center
Aurora, Colorado
720.848.0300
coloradocancercenter.org

University of Michigan
Comprehensive Cancer Center
Ann Arbor, Michigan
800.865.1125
mcancer.org

The University of Texas
MD Anderson Cancer Center
Houston, Texas
800.392.1611
mdanderson.org

Vanderbilt-Ingram Cancer Center
Nashville, Tennessee
800.811.8480
vicc.org

University of Wisconsin
Carbone Cancer Center
Madison, Wisconsin
608.265.1700
uwhealth.org/cancer

Yale Cancer Center/
Smilow Cancer Hospital
New Haven, Connecticut
855.4.SMILOW
yalecancercenter.org

My notes

Index

2nd opinion 94

21-gene RT-PCR test 45

biopsy 12, 17, 20–21, 26, 32, 34–36, 82–83

blood tests 17, 20, 26, 70, 82

breast-conserving therapy 30, 32, 38, 59, 77, 84–85, 94

breast reconstruction 12, 28, 31–32, 36–38, 91, 94

cancer stage 10, 34, 90

chemotherapy 12, 14, 32, 34, 40–54, 56, 66, 70, 85

clinical trial 10, 14, 58, 91

endocrine therapy 12–14, 32, 58–59, 66–74, 78, 80, 85

fertility 24

HER2 12, 14, 17, 22–23, 26, 32, 40–54, 56, 66, 83, 85

hereditary breast cancers 16–17, 24, 26, 82–83

hormone receptor 17, 22–23, 32, 44–45, 58–59, 66, 68–69, 74

imaging tests 18–21, 26, 32, 34–35, 77, 82–83, 94

immunohistochemistry 22

lumpectomy 12, 30–32, 36, 38, 58–59, 64, 77

lymph node 6–8, 10–12, 17–18, 21, 26, 28, 32, 34–35, 38, 44–47, 56, 58–61, 64, 68–69, 74, 78, 83–86

mammogram 17–19, 32, 77, 80

mastectomy 12, 30–32, 34, 36–38, 60–61, 64, 77, 84–85, 94

medical history 16–17, 26, 76–77, 80, 82–83

NCCN Member Institutions 107

NCCN Panel Members 106

nipple replacement 37

pathology report 20, 90, 94

physical exam 17, 20–21, 32, 34–35, 76–77, 80, 82–83

radiation therapy 12–14, 30, 38, 56–64, 66, 70, 77, 84–86

sentinel lymph node dissection 12, 38

supportive care 10

triple-negative breast cancer 44

Made in the USA
San Bernardino, CA
11 September 2018